Biomedical Engineering

Biomedical Engineering

Davon Matthews

hayle
medical

New York

Hayle Medical,
750 Third Avenue, 9ᵗʰ Floor,
New York, NY 10017, USA

Visit us on the World Wide Web at:
www.haylemedical.com

ISBN: 978-1-63241-547-9

Cataloging-in-Publication Data

Biomedical engineering / Davon Matthews.
   p. cm.
Includes bibliographical references and index.
ISBN 978-1-63241-547-9
1. Biomedical engineering. 2. Bioengineering. 3. Medicine. I. Matthews, Davon.
R856 .B56 2019
610.28--dc23

Table of Contents

Permissions

Index

Preface

The field concerned with the application of engineering for advancements in medicine and biology is known as biomedical engineering. It strives to develop solutions for healthcare issues so as to improve therapy, monitoring and diagnosis. It also involves equipment maintenance, testing, disposal and decommissioning. Prominent applications of biomedical engineering are the development of biocompatible prostheses, regenerative tissue growth, therapeutic and diagnostic medical devices, imaging technologies such as MRIs and ECGs, etc. This textbook is a compilation of chapters that discuss the most vital concepts in the field of biomedical engineering. Different approaches, evaluations and methodologies have been included herein. Coherent flow of topics, student-friendly language and extensive use of examples make this book an invaluable source of knowledge.

A detailed account of the significant topics covered in this book is provided below:

Chapter 1- Biomedical science is concerned with the diagnosis, treatment and prevention of diseases in humans. Biomedical engineering refers to the application of design concepts and engineering principles to the fields of medicine and biology for advancing healthcare. This is an introductory chapter, which will discuss in brief the various concepts and allied fields of biomedical science and biomedical engineering.

Chapter 2- Bioinformatics is a field of study, which is involved in the development of software tools and methods for understanding biological data. This chapter discusses the fundamental principles of bioinformatics, such as biodiversity informatics, gene prediction, structural bioinformatics, bioimage informatics, etc.

Chapter 3- Biomechanics is concerned with the study of biological systems, at all levels of organization from cell organelles to the organism level. This chapter closely examines the crucial concepts of biomechanics, such as statics, dynamics, kinematics and kinetics as well as the domains of nanobiomechanics, plant and sports biomechanics, among others.

Chapter 4- Any substance, which is engineered to interact with biological systems for therapeutic or diagnostic purposes, is called a biomaterial. The study of biomaterials is under the discipline of biomaterials science or biomaterials engineering. An understanding of biomaterials is facilitated by a study of biocompatibility, nanocellulose, cell encapsulation, etc. which have been extensively discussed in this chapter.

Chapter 5- Various devices and imaging techniques are integral to the field of biomedical engineering. A medical device is used for diagnosing a health condition and for the treatment and prevention of diseases. Medical imaging is a major area in medical devices. A detailed analysis of biomedical engineering devices and imaging techniques has been provided in this chapter, such as implant, prosthesis, tomography, image registration, radiology, radiomics, etc.

I would like to make a special mention of my publisher who considered me worthy of this opportunity and also supported me throughout the process. I would also like to thank the editing team at the back-end who extended their help whenever required.

Davon Matthews

Introduction to Biomedical Engineering

Biomedical science is concerned with the diagnosis, treatment and prevention of diseases in humans. Biomedical engineering refers to the application of design concepts and engineering principles to the fields of medicine and biology for advancing healthcare. This is an introductory chapter, which will discuss in brief the various concepts and allied fields of biomedical science and biomedical engineering.

Biomedical Science

Biomedical Science is the study of Life Science areas related to human health and disease.

Biomedical science serves medical science by allowing physicians to understand the critical processes associated with infectious diseases caused by bacteria, viruses, protozoans, and other microorganisms; the influence of body physiology and biochemistry on the maintenance of health; and the tolerance or immune-related rejection of transplanted tissues. It also offers a foundation to test a person's blood, urine, or tissue for the presence of disease and to develop new techniques to maintain health.

The legacy of biomedical science is long. Dutch scientist Antonio van Leeuwenhoek (1632–1723) first recognized the existence of cells in the fluids and tissues of the human body. Near the dawn of the nineteenth century, those observations allowed Robert Koch (1843–1910) to demonstrate the bacterial nature of diseases like anthrax, tuberculosis, and cholera. Physicians now understand that many types of bacteria cause disease, ranging from the relatively minor discomfort of gastrointestinal upset to the life-threatening release of toxins into the bloodstream, as in blood poisoning, or septicemia.

Viral diseases, including influenza, avian flu, human immunodeficiency virus (HIV/AIDS), Ebola viral hemorrhagic fever, rabies, and severe acute respiratory syndrome (SARS), also carry significant medical, social, political, and economic impacts. They hold the potential to reshape how modern society adapts to a shrinking global village.

Biomedical science is concerned with detecting diseases by a number of methods. In many diseases, like cancer, early detection can save a person's life. In this regard, the use of noninvasive imaging techniques such as positron emission spectroscopy (PET), magnetic resonance imaging (MRI), and computed tomography (CT) have allowed diagnosis without the need for exploratory surgery.

Biomedical Engineering

Biomedical engineering is a discipline that advances knowledge in engineering, biology and medicine, and improves human health through cross-disciplinary activities that integrate the engineering sciences with the biomedical sciences and clinical practice. It includes:

- The acquisition of new knowledge and understanding of living systems through the innovative and substantive application of experimental and analytical techniques based on the engineering sciences.

- The development of new devices, algorithms, processes and systems that advance biology and medicine and improve medical practice and health care delivery.

The term "biomedical engineering research" is thus defined in a broad sense: It includes not only the relevant applications of engineering to medicine but also to the basic life sciences.

As medical practice becomes more technologically based, a progressive shift is occurring in industry to meet the demand. Developments in science and engineering are increasingly being directed away from traditional technologies towards those required for health care in its widest sense. Although in many countries there is a problem with escalating costs in the medical sector, technology can contribute to economies because of falling costs of electronic/physics based components relative to those for personnel, and because of technologically based screening programmes.

Specialty Areas

Some of the well-established specialty areas within the field of biomedical engineering are bioinstrumentation, biomechanics, biomaterials, systems physiology, clinical engineering, and rehabilitation engineering.

Bioinstrumentation is the application of electronics and measurement principles and techniques to develop devices used in diagnosis and treatment of disease. Computers are becoming increasingly important in bioinstrumentation, from the microprocessor used to do a variety of small tasks in a single purpose instrument to the extensive computing power needed to process the large amount of information in a medical imaging system.

Biomechanics is mechanics applied to biological or medical problems. It includes the study of motion, of material deformation, of flow within the body and in devices, and transport of chemical constituents across biological and synthetic media and membranes. Efforts in biomechanics have developed the artificial heart and replacement heart valves, the artificial kidney, the artificial hip, as well as built a better understanding of the function of organs and musculoskeletal systems.

Biomaterials describe both living tissue and materials used for implantation. Understanding the properties of the living material is vital in the design of implant materials. The selection of an appropriate material to place in the human body may be one of the most difficult tasks faced by the biomedical engineer. Certain metal alloys, ceramics, polymers, and composites have been used as implantable materials. Biomaterials must be nontoxic, noncarcinogenic, chemically inert, stable, and mechanically strong enough to withstand the repeated forces of a lifetime.

Systems physiology is the term used to describe that aspect of biomedical engineering in which engineering strategies, techniques and tools are used to gain a comprehensive and integrated understanding of the function of living organisms ranging from bacteria to humans. Modeling is used in the analysis of experimental data and in formulating mathematical descriptions of physiological events. In research, models are used in designing new experiments to refine our knowledge. Living systems have highly regulated feedback control systems which can be examined in this way. Examples are the biochemistry of metabolism and the control of limb movements.

Clinical engineering is the application of technology for health care in hospitals. The clinical engineer is a member of the health care team along with physicians, nurses and other hospital staff. Clinical engineers are responsible for developing and maintaining computer databases of medical instrumentation and equipment records and for the purchase and use of sophisticated medical instruments. They may also work with physicians on projects to adapt instrumentation to the specific needs of the physician and the hospital. This often involves the interface of instruments with computer systems and customized software for instrument control and data analysis. Clinical engineers feel the excitement of applying the latest technology to health care.

Rehabilitation engineering is a new and growing specialty area of biomedical engineering. Rehabilitation engineers expand capabilities and improve the quality of life for individuals with physical impairments. Because the products of their labor are so personal, often developed for particular individuals or small groups, the rehabilitation engineer often works directly with the disabled individual.

These specialty areas frequently depend on each other. Often the biomedical engineer who works in an applied field will use knowledge gathered by biomedical engineers working in more basic areas. For example, the design of an artificial hip is greatly aided by a biomechanical study of the hip. The forces which are applied to the hip can be considered in the design and material selection for the prosthesis. Similarly, the design of systems to electrically stimulate paralyzed muscle to move in a controlled way uses knowledge of the behavior of the human musculoskeletal system. The selection of appropriate materials used in these devices falls within the realm of the biomaterials engineer. These are examples of the interactions among the specialty areas of biomedical engineering.

Neural Engineering

Neural engineering or neuroengineering in biomedicine is a discipline in which engineering technologies and mathematical and computational methods are combined with techniques in neuroscience and biology. Objectives of neural engineering include the enhancement of understanding of the functions of the human nervous system and the improvement of human performance, especially after injury or disease. The field is multidisciplinary in that it draws from the neurological sciences (especially neurobiology and neurology) as well as from a diverse range of engineering disciplines, including computer sciences, robotics, material sciences, signal processing, and systems modeling and simulation. The field covers a variety of subjects and applications; examples include brain-computer interfaces, neuroimaging, neuroinformatics, neural tissue engineering, and neurorobotics.

While the potential applications of neural engineering are broad, the discipline offers particular opportunities for improving motor and sensory function after major injury to the human central nervous system, such as that caused by stroke, traumatic brain injury, or spinal cord injury. For those conditions, new technologies can be applied to help reroute neural signals around damaged areas of the brain or spinal cord or to substitute one type of neural signal for another type that is lost after the injury.

Animal models that were developed in the field have enabled researchers to study recordings from various cortical areas during normal voluntary behaviors, which has provided insight into human neural pathways. Neural signals can be filtered and processed and then used to instruct computers, to control simple robotic devices, or to activate electrical stimulators to control limb muscles. Alternative approaches allow signals from skin or other sensory areas to be routed around damaged areas and to be delivered to the cerebral cortex by other means. For example, sensory signals from the eye or from skin can be detected by a range of electronic sensors and delivered to the cortex in the form of electrical stimulus trains.

Other developments in the field include advances in neural tissue engineering, which is aimed at the repair and regeneration of nerves; advances in neural recording systems that allow long-term recording from small groups of nerve fibers in peripheral muscle or skin nerves; and the development of implantable stimulators for use in promoting recovery of walking in individuals with spinal cord injury or for the restoration of motor function after cortical damage sustained as a result of stroke. For example, neural cuffs that are implanted around nerves innervating the foot sole can be used to sense foot contact during walking or to detect other phases of locomotion, allowing accurate programming of muscle nerve stimulation.

Bioinformatics

Bioinformatics involves the application of computer technology to manage volumes of biological information. Computers are used to not only store, but also gather, analyze and integrate biological and genetic data that can then be applied for such uses as gene-based drug discovery and development.

- Basic research: Bioinformatics is relied upon to assist with research into such areas as comparative and evolutionary genomics, functional genomics and genome wide association analysis. The mass of genomic data generated by high performance technologies has made this discipline vital for storing, managing and analyzing genomic information commonly used in biological research today.

- Biomedicine: The application of bioinformatics is proving quite useful in this field as the human genome has helped unlock the genetic components for many diseases. Potential applications include drug discovery, personalized medicine, preventative medicine and gene therapy.

- Microbiology: The potential applications here involve the study of microorganism genomes to assist with biotechnology developments, waste cleanup, climate change, antibiotic resistance and more.

- Agriculture: By sequencing the genomes of animals and plants, genetic knowledge can be gleaned to help produce stronger crops while improving the quality of livestock.

Biomechanics

Biomechanics is the science of movement of a living body, including how muscles, bones, tendons, and ligaments work together to produce movement. Biomechanics is part of the larger field of kinesiology, specifically focusing on the mechanics of movement. It is both a basic and applied science, encompassing research and practical use of its findings.

Biomechanics includes not only the structure of bones and muscles and the movement they can produce, but also the mechanics of blood circulation, renal function, and other body functions. Biomechanics represents the broad interplay between mechanics and biological systems. Biomechanics studies not only the human body but also animals and even extends to plants and the mechanical workings of cells.

Examples: The biomechanics of the squat includes consideration of the position and/or movement of the feet, hips, knees, back and shoulders and arms.

Elements of Biomechanics

- Statics: Studying systems that are in equilibrium, either at rest or moving at a constant velocity.

- Dynamics: Studying systems that are in motion with acceleration and deceleration.

- Kinematics: Describing the effect of forces on a system, motion patterns including linear and angular changes in velocity over time. Position, displacement, velocity, and acceleration are studied.

- Kinetics: Studying what causes motion, the forces and moments at work.

Biomaterial

A biomaterial is any matter, surface, or construct that interacts with biological systems. Biomaterials can be found/derived in nature and they can be also synthesized for different purposes in bioengineering and especially Tissue Engineering in Regenerative Medicine. The application is very wide. Regardless of the origin, they have to be biocompatible, since they will be used in replacing living tissues such as heart valves, hips (replacement), heart electrical impulse generator (pace makers), prostheses, etc. Minimal or absent immune response is to be expected. However, in many cases biomaterial is also requested to be biodegradable or bioresorbable in order to disappear from organism after fulfilling their function. Biomaterials are extensively developed and used in drug delivery systems as capsules or nanoshells, or microbasket for carrying drugs toward the target, and in scaffold biofabrication for supportive growth of particular tissues used in regenerative therapy.

Tissue Engineering

Tissue engineering evolved from the field of biomaterials development and refers to the practice of combining scaffolds, cells, and biologically active molecules into functional tissues. The goal of tissue engineering is to assemble functional constructs that restore, maintain, or improve damaged tissues or whole organs. Artificial skin and cartilage are examples of engineered tissues that have been approved by the FDA; however, current-ly they have limited use in human patients.

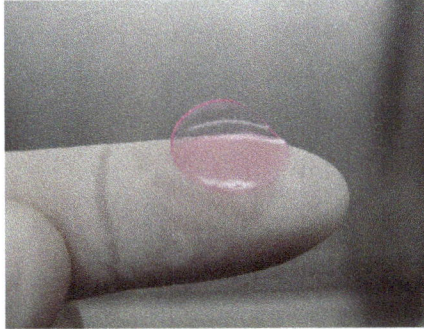

A mini bioengineered human liver that can be implanted into mice.

Regenerative medicine is a broad field that includes tissue engineering but also incor-porates research on self-healing – where the body uses its own systems, sometimes with help foreign biological material to recreate cells and rebuild tissues and organs. The terms "tissue engineering" and "regenerative medicine" have become largely inter-changeable, as the field hopes to focus on cures instead of treatments for complex, often chronic, diseases.

This field continues to evolve. In addition to medical applications, non-therapeu-tic applications include using tissues as biosensors to detect biological or chemical threat agents, and tissue chips that can be used to test the toxicity of an experimental medication.

Working of Tissue Engineering and Regenerative Medicine

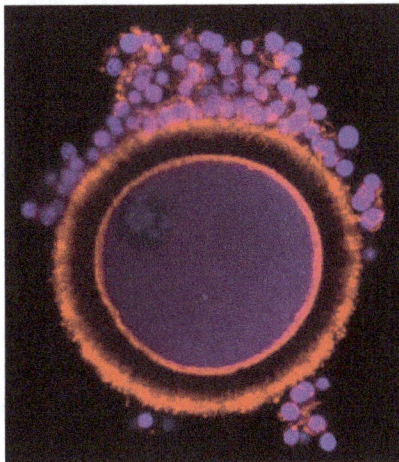

Cells are the building blocks of tissue, and tissues are the basic unit of function in the body. Generally, groups of cells make and secrete their own support structures, called extra-cellular matrix. This matrix, or scaffold, does more than just support the cells; it also acts as a relay station for various signaling molecules. Thus, cells receive messages from many sources that become available from the local environment. Each signal can start a chain of responses that determine what happens to the cell. By understanding how individual cells respond to signals, interact with their environment, and organize into tissues and organisms, researchers have been able to manipulate these processes to mend damaged tissues or even create new ones.

The process often begins with building a scaffold from a wide set of possible sources, from proteins to plastics. Once scaffolds are created, cells with or without a "cocktail" of growth factors can be introduced. If the environment is right, a tissue develops. In some cases, the cells, scaffolds, and growth factors are all mixed together at once, allowing the tissue to "self-assemble."

Another method to create new tissue uses an existing scaffold. The cells of a donor organ are stripped and the remaining collagen scaffold is used to grow new tissue. This process has been used to bioengineer heart, liver, lung, and kidney tissue. This approach holds great promise for using scaffolding from human tissue discarded during surgery and combining it with a patient's own cells to make customized organs that would not be rejected by the immune system.

The Way in Which Tissue Engineering and Regenerative Medicine Fit in with Current Medical Practices

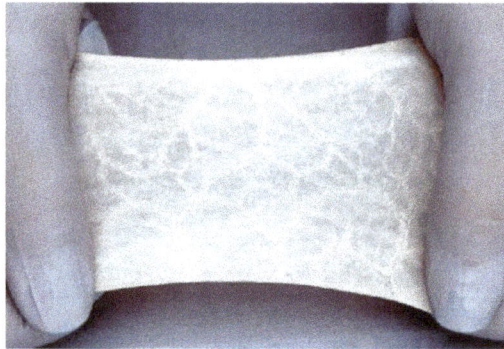

A biomaterial *made from pigs' intestines which can be used to heal wounds in humans. When moistened, the material, which is called SIS, is flexible and easy to handle.*

Currently, tissue engineering plays a relatively small role in patient treatment. Supplemental bladders, small arteries, skin grafts, cartilage, and even a full trachea have been implanted in patients, but the procedures are still experimental and very costly. While more complex organ tissues like heart, lung, and liver tissue have been successfully recreated in the lab, they are a long way from being fully reproducible and ready to implant into a patient. These tissues, however, can be quite useful in research, especially in drug development. Using functioning human tissue to help screen medication candidates could speed up development and provide key tools for facilitating personalized medicine while saving money and reducing the number of animals used for research.

Genetic Engineering

Genetic engineering is the artificial manipulation, modification, and recombination of DNA or other nucleic acid molecules in order to modify an organism or population of organisms.

Process And Techniques

Most recombinant DNA technology involves the insertion of foreign genes into the plasmids of common laboratory strains of bacteria. Plasmids are small rings of DNA; they are not part of the bacterium's chromosome (the main repository of the organism's genetic information). Nonetheless, they are capable of directing protein synthesis, and, like chromosomal DNA, they are reproduced and passed on to the bacterium's progeny. Thus, by incorporating foreign DNA (for example, a mammalian gene) into a bacterium, researchers can obtain an almost limitless number of copies of the inserted gene. Furthermore, if the inserted gene is operative (i.e., if it directs protein synthesis), the modified bacterium will produce the protein specified by the foreign DNA.

A subsequent generation of genetic engineering techniques that emerged in the early 21st century centered on gene editing. Gene editing, based on a technology known as CRISPR-Cas9, allows researchers to customize a living organism's genetic sequence by making very specific changes to its DNA. Gene editing has a wide array of applications, being used for the genetic modification of crop plants and livestock and of laboratory model organisms (e.g., mice). The correction of genetic errors associated with disease in animals suggests that gene editing has potential applications in gene therapy for humans.

Applications

Genetic engineering has advanced the understanding of many theoretical and practical aspects of gene function and organization. Through recombinant DNA techniques, bacteria have been created that are capable of synthesizing human insulin, human growth hormone, alpha interferon, a hepatitis B vaccine, and other medically useful substances. Plants may be genetically adjusted to enable them to fix nitrogen, and genetic diseases can possibly be corrected by replacing dysfunctional genes with normally functioning genes. Nevertheless, special concern has been focused on such achievements for fear that they might result in the introduction of unfavorable and possibly dangerous traits into microorganisms that were previously free of them—e.g., resistance to antibiotics, production of toxins, or a tendency to cause disease. Likewise, the application of gene editing in humans has raised ethical concerns, particularly regarding its potential use to alter traits such as intelligence and beauty.

References

- Biomedical-science, medical-magazines, science: encyclopedia.com, Retrieved 14 March 2018

- Neural-engineering, science: britannica.com, Retrieved 24 June 2018

- What-is-bioinformatics, key-concepts: usfhealthonline.com, Retrieved 28 March 2018

- Understanding-biomechanics-3498389: verywellfit.com, Retrieved 14 July 2018

- Tissue-engineering-and-regenerative-medicine, science-topics, science-education: nibib.nih.gov, Retrieved 17 June 2018

- Genetic-engineering, science: britannica.com, Retrieved 19 May 2018

Bioinformatics

Bioinformatics is a field of study, which is involved in the development of software tools and methods for understanding biological data. This chapter discusses the fundamental principles of bioinformatics, such as biodiversity informatics, gene prediction, structural bioinformatics, bioimage informatics, etc.

Bioinformatics is a hybrid science that links biological data with techniques for information storage, distribution, and analysis to support multiple areas of scientific research, including biomedicine. Bioinformatics is fed by high-throughput data-generating experiments, including genomic sequence determinations and measurements of gene expression patterns. Database projects curate and annotate the data and then distribute it via the World Wide Web. Mining these data leads to scientific discoveries and to the identification of new clinical applications. In the field of medicine in particular, a number of important applications for bioinformatics have been discovered. For example, it is used to identify correlations between gene sequences and diseases, to predict protein structures from amino acid sequences, to aid in the design of novel drugs, and to tailor treatments to individual patients based on their DNA sequences (pharmacogenomics).

The Data of Bioinformatics

The classic data of bioinformatics include DNA sequences of genes or full genomes; amino acid sequences of proteins; and three-dimensional structures of proteins, nucleic acids and protein–nucleic acid complexes. Additional "-omics" data streams include: transcriptomics, the pattern of RNA synthesis from DNA; proteomics, the distribution of proteins in cells; interactomics, the patterns of protein-protein and protein–nucleic acid interactions; and metabolomics, the nature and traffic patterns of transformations of small molecules by the biochemical pathways active in cells. In each case there is interest in obtaining comprehensive, accurate data for particular cell types and in identifying patterns of variation within the data. For example, data may fluctuate depending on cell type, timing of data collection (during the cell cycle, or diurnal, seasonal, or annual variations), developmental stage, and various external conditions. Metagenomics and metaproteomics extend these measurements to a comprehensive description of the organisms in an environmental sample, such as in a bucket of ocean water or in a soil sample.

Bioinformatics has been driven by the great acceleration in data-generation processes in biology. Genome sequencing methods show perhaps the most dramatic effects. In 1999 the nucleic acid sequence archives contained a total of 3.5 billion nucleotides, slightly more than the length of a single human genome; a decade later they contained more than 283 billion nucleotides, the length of about 95 human genomes.

Storage and Retrieval Of Data

In bioinformatics, data banks are used to store and organize data. Many of these entities collect DNA and RNA sequences from scientific papers and genome projects. Many databases are in the hands of international consortia. For example, an advisory committee made up of members of the European Molecular Biology Laboratory Nucleotide Sequence Database (EMBL-Bank) in the United Kingdom, the DNA Data Bank of Japan (DDBJ), and GenBank of the National Center for Biotechnology Information (NCBI) in the United States oversees the International Nucleotide Sequence Database Collaboration (INSDC). To ensure that sequence data are freely available, scientific journals require that new nucleotide sequences be deposited in a publicly accessible database as a condition for publication of an article. (Similar conditions apply to nucleic acid and protein structures.) There also exist genome browsers, databases that bring together all the available genomic and molecular information about a particular species.

The major database of biological macromolecular structure is the worldwide Protein Data Bank (wwPDB), a joint effort of the Research Collaboratory for Structural Bioinformatics (RCSB) in the United States, the Protein Data Bank Europe (PDBe) at the European Bioinformatics Institute in the United Kingdom, and the Protein Data Bank Japan at Ōsaka University. The homepages of the wwPDB partners contain links to the data files themselves, to expository and tutorial material (including news items), to facilities for deposition of new entries, and to specialized search software for retrieving structures.

Information retrieval from the data archives utilizes standard tools for identification of data items by keyword; for instance, one can type "aardvark myoglobin" into Google and retrieve the molecule's amino acid sequence. Other algorithms search data banks to detect similarities between data items. For example, a standard problem is to probe a sequence database with a gene or protein sequence of interest in order to detect entities with similar sequences.

Sequence Analysis

```
A5ASC3.1   14 SIKLWPPSQTTRLLLVERMANNLST..PSIFTRK..YGSLSKEEARENAKQIEEVACSTANQ.....HYEKEPDGDGGSAVQLYAKECSKLILEVLK 101
B4F917.1   13 SIKLWPPSESTRIMLVDRMTNNLST..ESIFSRK..YRLLGKQEAHENAKTIEELCFALADE.....HFREEPDGDGGSAVQLYAKETSKMMLEVLK 100
A9S1V2.1   23 VFKLWPPSQGTREAVRQKMALKLSS..ACFESQS..FARIELADAQEHARAIEEVAFGAAQE......ADSGGDKTGSAVVMVYAKHASKLMLETLR 109
B9GSN7.1   13 SVKLWPPSGQSTRLMLVERMTKNFIT..PSFISRK..YGLLSKEEAEEDAKKIEEVAFAAANQ.....HYEKQPDGDGGSSAVQIYAKESSRLMLEVLK 100
Q8HO56.1   30 SFSIWPPTQRTRDAVVRRLVDTLGG..DTILCKR..YGAVPAADAEPAARGIEAEAFDAAAA..SGEAAATASVEEGIKALQLYSKEVSRRLLDFVK 120
Q0D4Z3.2   44 SLSIWPPSQRTRDAVVRRLVQTLVA..PSILSQR..YGAVPEAEAGRAAAAVEAEAYAAVTES.SSAAAAPASVEDGIEVLQAYSKEVSRRLLELAK 135
B9MVW8.1   56 SFSIWPPTQRTRDAIISRLIETLST..TSVLSKR..YGTIPKEEASEASRRIEEEAFSGAST.......VASSEKDGLEVLQLYSKEISKRMLETVK 141
Q0IYC5.1   29 SFAVWPPTRRTRDAVVRRLVAVLSGDTTTALRKRYRYGAVPAADAERAARAVEAQAFDAASA....SSSSSSSVEDGIETLQLYSREVSNRLLAFVR 121
A9NWJ46.1  13 SIKLWPPSESTRLMLVERMTDNLSS..VSFFSRK..YGLLSKEEAAENAKRIEETAFLAAND....HEAKEPNLDDSSVVQFYAREASKLMLEALK 100
Q9C500.1   57 SLRIWPPTQKTRDAVLNRLIETLST..ESILSKR..YGTLKSDDATTVAKLIEEEAYGVASN.....AVSSDDDGIKILELYSKEISKRMLESVK 142
Q2HRI7.1   25 NYSIWPPKQRTRDAVKNRLIETLST..PSVLTKR..YGTMSADEASAAAIQIEDEAFSVANA.......SSSTSNDNVTILEVYSKEISKRMIETVK 110
Q9M7N3.1   28 SFKIWPPTQRTREAVVRRLVETLTS..QSVLSKR..YGVIPEEDATSAARIIEEEAFSVASV.ASAASTGGRPEDEWIEVLHIYSQEIXQRVVESAK 119
Q9M7N6.1   25 SFSIWPPTQRTRDAVINRLIESLST..PSILSKR..YGTLPQDEASETARLIEEEAFAAAGS.......TASDADDGIEILQVYSKEISKRMIDTVK 110
Q9LE82.1   14 SVKMWPPSKSTRLMLVERMTKNITT..PSIFSRK..YGLLSVEEAEQDAKRIEDLAFATANK.....HFQNEPDGDGTSAVHVYAKESSKLMLDVIK 101
Q9M651.2   13 SIKLWPPSLPTRKALIERITNNFSS..KTIFTEK..YGSLTKDQATENAKRIEDIAFSTANQ....QFEREPDGDGGSAVQLYAKECSKLILEVLK 100
B9R748.1   48 SLSIWPPTQRTRDAVITRLIETLSS..PSVLSKR..YGTISHDEAESAARRIEDEAFGVANT.......ATSAEDDGLEILQLYSKEISRRMLDTVK 133
```

The sequences of different genes or proteins may be aligned side-by-side to measure their similarity. This alignment compares protein sequences and genomic sequences containing WPP domains.

Since the Phage Φ-X174 was sequenced in 1977, the DNA sequences of thousands of organisms have been decoded and stored in databases. This sequence information is analyzed to determine genes that encode proteins, RNA genes, regulatory sequences, structural motifs, and repetitive sequences. A comparison of genes within a species or between different species can show similarities between protein functions, or relations between species (the use of molecular systematics to construct phylogenetic trees). With the growing amount of data, it long ago became impractical to analyze DNA sequences manually. Today, computer programs such as BLAST are used daily to search sequences from more than 260 000 organisms, containing over 190 billion nucleotides. These programs can compensate for mutations (exchanged, deleted or inserted bases) in the DNA sequence, to identify sequences that are related, but not identical. A variant of this sequence alignment is used in the sequencing process itself.

DNA Sequencing

Before sequences can be analyzed they have to be obtained. DNA sequencing is still a non-trivial problem as the raw data may be noisy or afflicted by weak signals. Algorithms have been developed for base calling for the various experimental approaches to DNA sequencing.

Sequence Assembly

Most DNA sequencing techniques produce short fragments of sequence that need to be assembled to obtain complete gene or genome sequences. The so-called shotgun sequencing technique (which was used, for example, by The Institute for Genomic Research (TIGR) to sequence the first bacterial genome, *Haemophilus influenzae*) generates the sequences of many thousands of small DNA fragments (ranging from 35 to 900 nucleotides long, depending on the sequencing technology). The ends of these fragments overlap and, when aligned properly by a genome assembly program, can be used to reconstruct the complete genome. Shotgun sequencing yields sequence data quickly, but the task of assembling the fragments can be quite complicated for larger genomes. For a genome as large as the human genome, it may take many days of CPU time on large-memory, multiprocessor computers to assemble the fragments, and the resulting assembly usually contains numerous gaps that must be filled in later. Shotgun sequencing is the method of choice for virtually all genomes sequenced today, and genome assembly algorithms are a critical area of bioinformatics research.

Genome Annotation

In the context of genomics, annotation is the process of marking the genes and other biological features in a DNA sequence. This process needs to be automated because most genomes are too large to annotate by hand, not to mention the desire to annotate as many genomes as possible, as the rate of sequencing has ceased to pose a bottleneck.

Annotation is made possible by the fact that genes have recognizable start and stop regions, although the exact sequence found in these regions can vary between genes.

The first description of a comprehensive genome annotation system was published in 1995 by the team at The Institute for Genomic Research that performed the first complete sequencing and analysis of the genome of a free-living organism, the bacterium *Haemophilus influenzae*. Owen White designed and built a software system to identify the genes encoding all proteins, transfer RNAs, ribosomal RNAs (and other sites) and to make initial functional assignments. Most current genome annotation systems work similarly, but the programs available for analysis of genomic DNA, such as the Gene-Mark program trained and used to find protein-coding genes in *Haemophilus influenzae*, are constantly changing and improving.

Following the goals that the Human Genome Project left to achieve after its closure in 2003, a new project developed by the National Human Genome Research Institute in the U.S appeared. The so-called ENCODE project is a collaborative data collection of the functional elements of the human genome that uses next-generation DNA-sequencing technologies and genomic tiling arrays, technologies able to automatically generate large amounts of data at a dramatically reduced per-base cost but with the same accuracy (base call error) and fidelity (assembly error).

Computational Evolutionary Biology

Evolutionary biology is the study of the origin and descent of species, as well as their change over time. Informatics has assisted evolutionary biologists by enabling researchers to:

- Trace the evolution of a large number of organisms by measuring changes in their DNA, rather than through physical taxonomy or physiological observations alone.

- More recently, compare entire genomes, which permits the study of more complex evolutionary events, such as gene duplication, horizontal gene transfer, and the prediction of factors important in bacterial speciation.

- Build complex computational population genetics models to predict the outcome of the system over time.

- Track and share information on an increasingly large number of species and organisms.

Future work endeavors to reconstruct the now more complex tree of life.

The area of research within computer science that uses genetic algorithms is sometimes confused with computational evolutionary biology, but the two areas are not necessarily related.

Comparative Genomics

The core of comparative genome analysis is the establishment of the correspondence between genes (orthology analysis) or other genomic features in different organisms. It is these intergenomic maps that make it possible to trace the evolutionary processes responsible for the divergence of two genomes. A multitude of evolutionary events acting at various organizational levels shape genome evolution. At the lowest level, point mutations affect individual nucleotides. At a higher level, large chromosomal segments undergo duplication, lateral transfer, inversion, transposition, deletion and insertion. Ultimately, whole genomes are involved in processes of hybridization, polyploidization and endosymbiosis, often leading to rapid speciation. The complexity of genome evolution poses many exciting challenges to developers of mathematical models and algorithms, who have recourse to a spectrum of algorithmic, statistical and mathematical techniques, ranging from exact, heuristics, fixed parameter and approximation algorithms for problems based on parsimony models to Markov chain Monte Carlo algorithms for Bayesian analysis of problems based on probabilistic models.

Many of these studies are based on the detection of sequence homology to assign sequences to protein families.

Pan Genomics

Pan genomics is a concept introduced in 2005 by Tettelin and Medini which eventually took root in bioinformatics. Pan genome is the complete gene repertoire of a particular taxonomic group: although initially applied to closely related strains of a species, it can be applied to a larger context like genus, phylum etc. It is divided in two parts- The Core genome: Set of genes common to all the genomes under study (These are often housekeeping genes vital for survival) and The Dispensable/Flexible Genome: Set of genes not present in all but one or some genomes under study. A bioinformatics tool BPGA can be used to characterize the Pan Genome of bacterial species.

Genetics of Disease

With the advent of next-generation sequencing we are obtaining enough sequence data to map the genes of complex diseases such as diabetes, infertility, breast cancer or Alzheimer's Disease. Genome-wide association studies are a useful approach to pinpoint the mutations responsible for such complex diseases. Through these studies, thousands of DNA variants have been identified that are associated with similar diseases and traits. Furthermore, the possibility for genes to be used at prognosis, diagnosis or treatment is one of the most essential applications. Many studies are discussing both the promising ways to choose the genes to be used and the problems and pitfalls of using genes to predict disease presence or prognosis.

Analysis of Mutations in Cancer

In cancer, the genomes of affected cells are rearranged in complex or even unpredictable ways. Massive sequencing efforts are used to identify previously unknown point mutations in a variety of genes in cancer. Bioinformaticians continue to produce specialized automated systems to manage the sheer volume of sequence data produced, and they create new algorithms and software to compare the sequencing results to the growing collection of human genome sequences and germline polymorphisms. New physical detection technologies are employed, such as oligonucleotide microarrays to identify chromosomal gains and losses (called comparative genomic hybridization), and single-nucleotide polymorphism arrays to detect known *point mutations*. These detection methods simultaneously measure several hundred thousand sites throughout the genome, and when used in high-throughput to measure thousands of samples, generate terabytes of data per experiment. Again the massive amounts and new types of data generate new opportunities for bioinformaticians. The data is often found to contain considerable variability, or noise, and thus Hidden Markov model and change-point analysis methods are being developed to infer real copy number changes.

Two important principles can be used in the analysis of cancer genomes bioinformatically pertaining to the identification of mutations in the exome. First, cancer is a disease of accumulated somatic mutations in genes. Second cancer contains driver mutations which need to be distinguished from passengers.

With the breakthroughs that this next-generation sequencing technology is providing to the field of Bioinformatics, cancer genomics could drastically change. These new methods and software allow bioinformaticians to sequence many cancer genomes quickly and affordably. This could create a more flexible process for classifying types of cancer by analysis of cancer driven mutations in the genome. Furthermore, tracking of patients while the disease progresses may be possible in the future with the sequence of cancer samples.

Another type of data that requires novel informatics development is the analysis of lesions found to be recurrent among many tumors.

Gene and Protein Expression

Analysis of Gene Expression

The expression of many genes can be determined by measuring mRNA levels with multiple techniques including microarrays, expressed cDNA sequence tag (EST) sequencing, serial analysis of gene expression (SAGE) tag sequencing, massively parallel signature sequencing (MPSS), RNA-Seq, also known as "Whole Transcriptome Shotgun Sequencing" (WTSS), or various applications of multiplexed in-situ hybridization. All of these techniques are extremely noise-prone and/or subject to bias in the biological measurement, and a major research area in computational biology involves developing statistical tools to separate signal from noise in high-throughput gene expression studies. Such studies are often used to determine the genes implicated in a disorder: one might compare microarray data from cancerous epithelial cells to data from non-cancerous cells to determine the transcripts that are up-regulated and down-regulated in a particular population of cancer cells.

Analysis of Protein Expression

Protein microarrays and high throughput (HT) mass spectrometry (MS) can provide a snapshot of the proteins present in a biological sample. Bioinformatics is very much involved in making sense of protein microarray and HT MS data; the former approach faces similar problems as with microarrays targeted at mRNA, the latter involves the problem of matching large amounts of mass data against predicted masses from protein sequence databases, and the complicated statistical analysis of samples where multiple, but incomplete peptides from each protein are detected. Cellular protein localization in a tissue context can be achieved through affinity proteomics displayed as spatial data based on immunohistochemistry and tissue microarrays.

Analysis of Regulation

Regulation is the complex orchestration of events by which a signal, potentially an extracellular signal such as a hormone, eventually leads to an increase or decrease in the activity of one or more proteins. Bioinformatics techniques have been applied to explore various steps in this process.

For example, gene expression can be regulated by nearby elements in the genome. Promoter analysis involves the identification and study of sequence motifs in the DNA surrounding the coding region of a gene. These motifs influence the extent to which that region is transcribed into mRNA. Enhancer elements far away from the promoter can also regulate gene expression, through three-dimensional looping interactions. These interactions can be determined by bioinformatic analysis of chromosome conformation capture experiments.

Expression data can be used to infer gene regulation: one might compare microarray data from a wide variety of states of an organism to form hypotheses about the genes involved in each state. In a single-cell organism, one might compare stages of the cell cycle, along with various stress conditions (heat shock, starvation, etc.). One can then apply clustering algorithms to that expression data to determine which genes are co-expressed. For example, the upstream regions (promoters) of co-expressed genes can be searched for over-represented regulatory elements. Examples of clustering algorithms applied in gene clustering are k-means clustering, self-organizing maps (SOMs), hierarchical clustering, and consensus clustering methods.

Analysis of Cellular Organization

Several approaches have been developed to analyze the location of organelles, genes, proteins, and other components within cells. This is relevant as the location of these components affects the events within a cell and thus helps us to predict the behavior of biological systems. A gene ontology category, *cellular compartment*, has been devised to capture subcellular localization in many biological databases.

Microscopy and Image Analysis

Microscopic pictures allow us to locate both organelles as well as molecules. It may also help us to distinguish between normal and abnormal cells, e.g. in cancer.

Protein Localization

The localization of proteins helps us to evaluate the role of a protein. For instance, if a protein is found in the nucleus it may be involved in gene regulation or splicing. By contrast, if a protein is found in mitochondria, it may be involved in respiration or other metabolic processes. Protein localization is thus an important component of protein function prediction. There are well developed protein subcellular localization prediction resources available, including protein subcellualr location databases, and prediction tools.

Nuclear Organization of Chromatin

Data from high-throughput chromosome conformation capture experiments, such as Hi-C (experiment) and ChIA-PET, can provide information on the spatial proximity of DNA loci. Analysis of these experiments can determine the three-dimensional structure and nuclear organization of chromatin. Bioinformatic challenges in this field include partitioning the genome into domains, such as Topologically Associating Domains (TADs), that are organised together in three-dimensional space.

Network and Systems Biology

Network analysis seeks to understand the relationships within biological networks such as metabolic or protein–protein interaction networks. Although biological networks can be constructed from a single type of molecule or entity (such as genes), network biology often attempts to integrate many different data types, such as proteins, small molecules, gene expression data, and others, which are all connected physically, functionally, or both.

Systems biology involves the use of computer simulations of cellular subsystems (such as the networks of metabolites and enzymes that comprise metabolism, signal transduction pathways and gene regulatory networks) to both analyze and visualize the complex connections of these cellular processes. Artificial life or virtual evolution attempts to understand evolutionary processes via the computer simulation of simple (artificial) life forms.

Molecular Interaction Networks

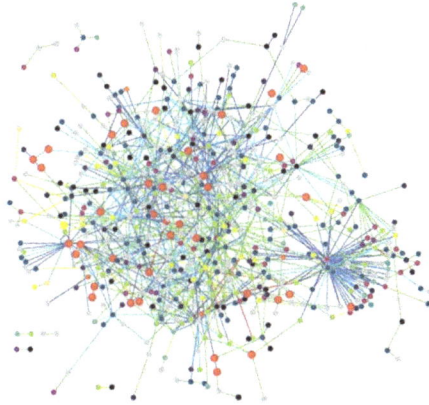

Interactions between proteins are frequently visualized and analyzed using networks. This network is made up of protein–protein interactions from *Treponema pallidum*, the causative agent of syphilis and other diseases.

Tens of thousands of three-dimensional protein structures have been determined by X-ray crystallography and protein nuclear magnetic resonance spectroscopy (protein NMR) and a central question in structural bioinformatics is whether it is practical to predict possible protein–protein interactions only based on these 3D shapes, without performing protein–protein interaction experiments. A variety of methods have been developed to tackle the protein–protein docking problem, though it seems that there is still much work to be done in this field.

Other interactions encountered in the field include Protein–ligand (including drug) and protein–peptide. Molecular dynamic simulation of movement of atoms about rotatable bonds is the fundamental principle behind computational algorithms, termed docking algorithms, for studying molecular interactions.

Gene Prediction

Gene prediction is one of the most important and alluring problems in computational biology. Its importance comes from the inherent value of the set of protein-coding genes for other analysis. Its allure is based on the apparently simple rules that the transcriptional machinery uses: strong, easily recognizable signals within the genome such as open reading frames, consensus splice sites and nearly universal start and stop codon sequences. These signals are highly conserved, are relatively easy to model, and have been the focus of a number of algorithms trying to locate all the protein-coding genes in a genome using only the sequence of one or more genomes. This technique, so-called *de novo* prediction, does not use information about expressed sequences such as proteins or mRNAs.

Gene Prediction Methods

There are mainly two classes of methods for computational gene prediction. One is based on sequence similarity searches, while the other is gene structure and signal-based searches, which is also referred to as *ab initio* gene finding.

Sequence Similarity Searches

Sequence similarity search is a conceptually simple approach that is based on finding similarity in gene sequences between ESTs (expressed sequence tags), proteins, or other genomes to the input genome. This approach is based on the assumption that functional regions (exons) are more conserved evolutionarily than nonfunctional regions (intergenic or intronic regions). Once there is similarity between a certain genomic region and an EST, DNA, or protein, the similarity information can be used to infer gene structure or function of that region. EST-based sequence similarity usually has drawbacks in that ESTs only correspond to small portions of the gene sequence, which means that it is often difficult to predict the complete gene structure of a given region.

Local alignment and global alignment are two methods based on similarity searches. The most common local alignment tool is the BLAST family of programs, which detects sequence similarity to known genes, proteins, or ESTs. Two more types of software, PROCRUSTES and GeneWise, use global alignment of a homologous protein to translated ORFs in a genomic sequence for gene prediction. A new heuristic method based on pairwise genome comparison has been implemented in the software called CSTfinder. The biggest limitation to this type of approaches is that only about half of the genes being discovered have significant homology to genes in the databases.

Ab initio Gene Prediction Methods

The second class of methods for the computational identification of genes is to use gene structure as a template to detect genes, which is also called *ab initio* prediction. *Ab initio* gene predictions rely on two types of sequence information: signal sensors and content sensors. Signal sensors refer to short sequence motifs, such as splice sites, branch points, polypyrimidine tracts, start codons and stop codons. Exon detection must rely on the content sensors, which refer to the patterns of codon usage that are unique to a species, and allow coding sequences to be distinguished from the surrounding non-coding sequences by statistical detection algorithms.

Many algorithms are applied for modeling gene structure, such as Dynamic Programming, linear discriminant analysis, Linguist methods, Hidden Markov Model and

Neural Network. Based on these models, a great number of *ab initio* gene prediction programs have been developed.

In Hidden Markov Model, transitions between sub-models corresponding to particular gene components are modeled as unobserved ("hidden") Markov processes, which determine the probability of generating particular (observable) nucleotides. Since exon and intron lengths appear to be constrained by factors related to pre-mRNA splicing, and do not exhibit geometric distributions, a more general model is required to accurately account for the lengths of exons and introns in real genes. So a Generalized Hidden Markov Model (GHMM) is developed, in which subsequent states are generated according to a Markov chain but have arbitrary (instead of fixed unit) length distributions. Figure given below illustrates the state transition in eukaryotic genomic sequences.

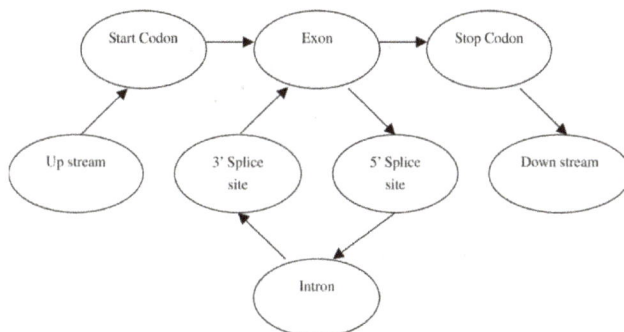

Figure: State transition of HMM modeling eukaryotic genes.

Suppose we are given a DNA sequence S of length L and a parse ϕ also of length L. The conditional probability of the parse ϕ, given that the sequence generated is S, can be computed using Bayes' Rule as:

$$P\{\phi \mid S\} = \frac{P\{\phi, S\}}{\sum\limits_{\psi \in \phi L} P\{\psi, S\}}$$

Here, ϕL is the set of all parses of length L. Now, given a particular DNA sequence S, we can find a parse ϕL that maximizes the likelihood of generating. In other words, for a particular sequence, we can find the functional unit (for example, the promoter region) that the sequence is most likely to represent. Thus, the model can be used for automatic annotation of DNA sequences.

Other Methods

The major limitation with HMM method is that we have a little knowledge of gene structures, especially for new sequencing genomes. Furthermore, current set of known genes is limited and certainly does not represent all potential gene features or their organizational themes. So recently some techniques in physics and signal processing have been applied to recognize genes.

It is well known that base sequences in the protein-coding regions of DNA molecules have a period-3 component because of the codon structure involved in the translation of base sequences into amino acids. Discrete Fourier Transform (DFT) is suitable for processing periodicity. For a DNA sequence of length N, assume $u_A(n), u_T(n), u_C(n),$ and $u_G(n)$, which represent the binary indicator function for the corresponding nucleotide. It takes the value 1 at index n if the corresponding nucleotide is present at that position, and takes the value 0 otherwise. Applying DFT to each of these sequences produces four spectral representations, represented as $U_A(k), U_T(k), U_C(k),$ and $U_G(k)$, respectively. The total frequency spectrum of the given DNA sequence is defined as:

$$S(k) = |U_A(k)|^2 + |U_T(k)|^2 + |U_C(k)|^2 + |U_G(k)|^2$$

In coding regions of DNA, S(k) typically has a peak at the frequency $k = N/3$, whereas in noncoding regions, it generally does not have any significant peaks. By this property, gene predictor can be constructed.

Issues in Gene Prediction

Three types of posttranscriptional events influence the translation of mRNA into protein and the accuracy of gene prediction. First, the genetic code of a given genome may vary from the universal code. Second, one tissue may splice a given mRNA differently from another, thus creating two similar but also partially different mRNAs encoding two related but different proteins. Third, mRNAs may be edited, changing the sequence of the mRNA and, as a result, of the encoded protein. Such changes also depend on interaction of RNA with RNA-binding proteins. Then there are issues of frame-shifts, insertions and deletions of bases, overlapping genes, genes on the complementary strand etc. Straight-forward solutions therefore do not work when we need to take all these issues into considerations.

Gene Prediction in Prokaryotes

Understanding Prokaryotic Gene Structure

The knowledge of gene structure is very important when we set out to solve the problem of gene prediction. The gene structure of Prokaryotes can be captured in terms of the following characteristics.

Promoter Elements

The process of gene expression begins with transcription - the making of an mRNA copy of a gene by an RNA polymerase. Prokaryotic RNA polymerases are actually assemblies of several different proteins (alpha, beta and beta-prime) that each play a distinct and important role in the functioning of the enzyme. The -35 and -10 sequences recognized by any particular sigma factor are usually described as a consensus sequence - essentially the set of most commonly found nucleotides at the equivalent positions of other genes that are transcribed by RNA polymerases containing the same sigma factor.

Open Reading Frames

Since stop codons are found in uninformative nucleotide sequences, approximately once every 21 codons (3 out of 64), a run of 30 or more triplet codons that does not include a stop codon is in itself a good evidence that the region corresponds to the coding sequence of a prokaryotic gene. One hallmark of prokaryotic genes that is related to their translation is the presence of the set of sequences around which ribosomes assemble at the 5' end of each open reading frame. Often found immediately downstream of transcriptional sites and just upstream of the first start codon, ribosome loading sites sequences almost invariably include the nucleotide sequence 5'-AGGAGGU-3'.

Termination Sequences

Just as the RNA polymerases begin transcription at recognizable transcriptional start sites immediately downstream from promoters, the vast majority of prokaryotic operons also contain specific signals for the termination of transcription called intrinsic terminators. Intrinsic terminators have two prominent structural features 1) a sequence of nucleotides that include an inverted repeat and 2) a run of roughly six uracils immediately following the inverted repeats.

Our Solution

HMMs have been used to analyze DNA, to model certain protein-binding sites in DNA and in protein analysis. The HMM models we use to find genes in E.Coli. range from simple models based on one-to-one correspondence between the codons and the HMM states to more complex HMMs with states corresponding to amino acids and intergenic regions.

In addition to the above HMM models, we have developed a Neural Networks to classify a set of nucleotide sequences into protein-encoding genes and non-coding regions.

Hidden Markov Model 1

The model is characterized by the following:

The number of states in the model : Although the states are hidden, for many practical applications there is often some physical significance attached to the states or to sets of states of the model. In our case, the states may be divided in three classes - one state for the start codon, one state for the stop codon, and a set of 59 states for the rest of the intragenic codons.

The number of distinct observation symbols per state : The start state has two observation symbols, each corresponding to a start codon, namely ATG and GTG. The stop state has three observation symbols corresponding to three stop codons, namely TAG, TAA and TGA. Finally, each state belonging to the set of 59 states has one observation symbol, each corresponding to one codon out of the remaining of the 64 possible codons.

State transition probability distribution: Transitions are initialized to every state from every other state, except for the stop state. In case of stop state, transitions only happen into the state but not out of the state. The initialization of state transition probabilities is on a random basis with the only constraint that the sum of probabilities of all the transitions going out of a state is 1.

Observation symbol probability distribution: The observation symbol probabilities are also initialized randomly in case of start and stop states. In case of the rest of 59 states, each state has only one observation symbol, so the observation symbol probability is set to 1.

Initial state distribution : Only the start state is allowed an initial state probability (= 1) and no other state is allowed to do so.

This model is then trained using a set of genes extracted from a part of the annotated genome. The training is done using Baum-Welch algorithm for HMMs. The trained HMM is then used to calculate the normalized logarithmic probability for a given sequence to be a gene.

(Extended HMM 1)This same model is then extended to take a genome sequence (or part of a genome sequence) as input and annotate it with gene information. This is done by adding an extra state that corresponds to the intergenic region. The state transition probability table is then extended so that there is transition into the IR state (intergenic region state) from the stop state and there is transition from the IR state into the start state and the IR state itself. These probabilities are randomly initialized. Also, all 64 possible codons are observation symbols for the IR state and their probabilities are randomly initialized. The initial state distribution is modified to include IR region apart from start state and their probabilities are initialized as 0.01 and 0.99 respectively. This model is then trained using a part of the annotated genome sequence. The trained model is then used to annotate the genome using Viterbi algorithm.

Hidden Markov Model 2

The model is characterized by the following:

The number of states in the model : The states may be divided into three sets - one state for the start codon, one state for the stop codon, and a set of 20 states each standing for an amino acid.

The number of distinct observation symbols per state : The start state has two obser-vation symbols, each corresponding to a start codon, namely ATG and GTG. The stop state has three observation symbols corresponding to three stop codons, namely TAG, TAA and TGA. Finally, each state (remember each state corresponds to one amino acid) belonging to the set of 20 states has as observation symbols all codons that translate into that amino acid. For example, the state corresponding to Glycine in the model has GGA, GGG, GGC and GGT as its observation symbols.

- State transition probability distribution : As in the case of HM Model 1, tran-sitions are initialized to every state from every other state, except for the stop state. In case of stop state, transitions only happen into the state but not out of the state. The initializations of state transition probabilities is on a random basis with the only constraint that the sum of probabilities of all the transitions going out of a state is 1.

- Observation symbol probability distribution : The observation symbol proba-bilities are also initialized randomly.

- Initial state distribution : Only the start state is allowed an initial state probabil-ity (= 1) and no other state is allowed to do so.

This model is then trained using a set of genes extracted from a part of the annotated genome. The training is done using Baum-Welch algorithm for HMMs. The trained HMM is then used to calculate the normalized logarithmic probability for a given se-quence to be a gene.

(Extended HMM 2)This same model is then extended to take a genome sequence (or part of a genome sequence) as input and annotate it with gene information. This is done in a fashion similar to HMModel 1.

Neural Networks

In addition to the above HMM models, we have developed an ANN to classify a set of nucleotide sequences into protein-encoding genes and non-coding regions. The search involves two steps - a sequence encoding step to convert genes into neural network in-put vectors and a neural network classification step to map input vectors to appropriate classes (i.e. coding or non-coding).

- Architecture: The ANN is a three layer network with one input layer, on hidden layer and one output layer. The input layer has 70 input nodes, out of which 64 correspond to all possible codons, 4 correspond to the nucleotides themselves (i.e. A, T, G and C), and two for chemically similar nulceotides - purines (A, T) and pyrimidines (G, C). The number of nodes in the hidden layer is randomly set to 20, and the number of output layer nodes is set to 2 (corresponding to two classes of sequences, coding and noncoding).

Input vector encoding: The encoding of input sequence into neural network input vector is done using ngrams. An ngram is a vector of nodes. Each node corresponds to a parameter, and its value is the normalized frequency of occurance of that parameter in the input sequence. For example, the node corresponding to the codon 'ACG' contains the number of occurrences of ACG divided by the total number of codons in the given sequence, as its value. Similarly, the node corresponding to 'A' contains the total number of occurrences of A in the input sequence divided by the length of the input sequence. The node for pyrines contains the total number of occurrences of A and T together in the sequence, and so on.

The ANN classification employs three-layered, feed-forward, back-propagation network. This ANN is trained using a pre-classified set of sequences consisting of both coding and non-coding sequences. The trained ANN is then used for classification.

Structural Bioinformatics

Structural Bioinformatics is generally looked as a branch of bioinformatics mainly about problems of structural biology, which the word "structural" is referred to here. In the early days, it was also named as "computational structural biology", using the distinctive techniques of computational molecular simulations. And the research interests were mainly focused in analysis and prediction of the three dimensional structures and related functions of biological macromolecules such as proteins, RNA, and DNA.

However, the fast developments in technologies and combinations with other fields make structural bioinformatics more and more diverse and interdisciplinary. Mathematics, statistics, informational sciences, bioinformatics, biophysics, computational chemistry, structural biology, enzymology, medical engineering, pharmaceutical sciences, and much more other disciplines are making contributions to structural bioinformatics. In the meanwhile, its applications are expanding into much more fields, like comparisons of overall folds and local motifs of both primary, secondary and tertiary structures, structural and functional predictions, molecular mechanism of folding/unfolding of macromolecules, evolution and bioengineering, binding interactions in the macromolecules complexes like drug-target complex, molecular mechanism of enzymatic catalysis, as well as other structure-function relationships. In addition to its wide application in the researches of biological sciences, it is showing more power in the industries of bioengineering and drug developments.

Application of Structural Bioinformatics in Drug Design

Drug design is always one of the focuses of applications in structural biology and biochemistry. The burst of computational power boost the emergence of a diversity of new sciences and technologies, including structural bioinformatics. Logically, it is quickly applied into the discovery and design of new drugs, such as the in silico structural or functional analyses on the target proteins, the virtual screening of drug candidates, constructions of databases and drug-target interaction networks, and so on. The applications of the new methods of structural bioinformatics are often surprising and interesting.

Bioimage Informatics

Bioimage informatics employs computational and statistical techniques to analyze images and related metadata. Bioimage informatics approaches are useful in a number of applications, such as measuring the effects of drugs on cells , localizing cellular proteomes , tracking of cellular motion and activity , mapping of gene expression in developing embryos and adult brains , and many others. Traditionally, bioimage analysis has been done by visual inspection, but this is tedious and error-prone. Results from visual analysis are not easily compared between papers or groups. Furthermore, as bioimage data is increasingly used to understand gene function on a genome scale, datasets of subtle phenotype changes are becoming too large for manual analysis. For example, it is estimated that having a single image for every combination of cell type, protein, and timescale would require on the order of 100 billion images . Over the past fourteen years, the traditional visual, knowledge-capture approach has begun to be replaced with automated, data-driven approaches.

Data Modalities

Several data collection systems and platforms are used, which require different methods to be handled optimally.

Fluorescent Microscopy

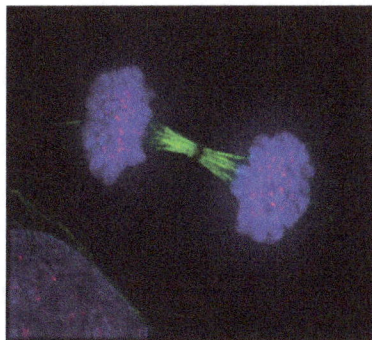

Figure: Fluorescent image of a cell in telophase. Multiple dyes were imaged and are shown in different colors.

Fluorescent microscopy allows the direct visualization of molecules at the subcellular level, in both live and fixed cells. Molecules of interest are marked with either green fluorescent protein (GFP), another fluorescent protein, or a fluorescently-labeled antibody. Several types of microscope are regularly used: widefield, confocal, or two-photon. Most microscopy system will also support the collection of time-series (movies).

In general, filters are used so that each dye is imaged separately (for example, a blue filter is used to image Hoechst, and then rapidly switched to a green filter to image GFP). For consumption, the images are often displayed in false color by showing each channel in a different color, but these may not even be related to the original wavelengths used. In some cases, the original image could even have been acquired in non-visible wavelengths (infrared is common).

The choices at the image acquisition stage will influence the analysis and often require special processing. Confocal stacks will require 3D processing and widefield pseudo-stacks will often benefit from digital deconvolution to remove the out-of-focus light.

The advent of automated microscopes that can acquire many images automatically is one of the reasons why analysis cannot be done by eye (otherwise, annotation would rapidly become the research bottleneck). Using automated microscopes means that some images might be out-of-focus (automated focus finding systems may sometimes be incorrect), contain a small number of cells, or be filled with debris. Therefore, the images generated will be harder to analyze than images acquired by an operator as they would have chosen other locations to image and focus correctly. On the other hand, the operator might introduce an unconscious bias in his selection by choosing only the cells whose phenotype is most like the one expected before the experiment.

Histology

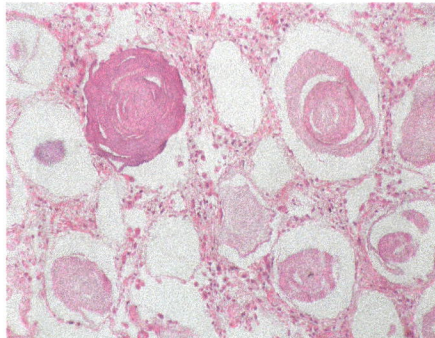

A histology image of alveolar microlithiasis

Histology is a microscopy application where tissue slices are stained and observed under the microscope (typically light microscope, but electron microscopy is also used).

When using a light microscope, unlike the case of fluorescent imaging, images are typically acquired using standard color camera-systems. This reflects partially the history of the field, where humans were often interpreting the images, but also the fact that the sample can be illuminated with white light and all light collected rather than having to excite fluorophores. When more than one dye is used, a necessary preprocessing step is to unmix the channels and recover an estimate of the pure dye-specific intensities.

It has been shown that the subcellular location of stained proteins can be identified from histology images.

If the goal is a medical diagnostic, then histology applications will often fall into the realm of digital pathology or automated tissue image analysis, which are sister fields of bioimage informatics. The same computational techniques are often applicable, but the goals are medically- rather than research-oriented.

Important Problems

Subcellular Location Analysis

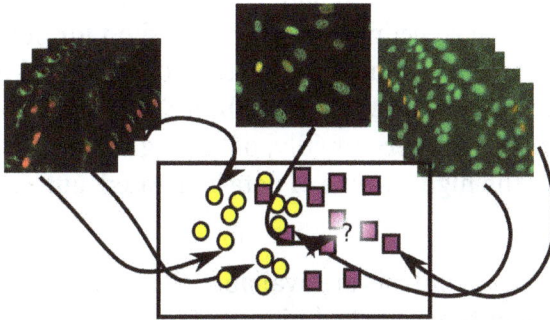

Figure: Subcellular Location Example. Examples of different patterns are mapped into a two-dimensional space by computing different image features. Image of unknown proteins are similarly mapped into this space and a nearest neighbor search or other classifier can be used for assigning a location to this unclassified protein.

Subcellular location analysis was one of the initial problems in this field. In its supervised mode, the problem is to learn a classifier that can recognize images from the major cell organelles based on images.

Methods used are based on machine learning, building a discriminative classifier based on numeric features computed from the image. Features are either generic features from computer vision, such as Haralick texture features or features specially designed to capture biological factors (e.g., co-localization with a nuclear marker being a typical example).

For the basic problem of identifying organelles, very high accuracy values can be obtained, including better than results. These methods are useful in basic cell biology research, but have also been applied to the discovery of proteins whose location changes in cancer cells.

However, classification into organelles is a limited form of the problem as many proteins will localize to multiple locations simultaneously (mixed patterns) and many patterns can be distinguished even though they are not different membrane-bound components. There are several unsolved problems in this area and research is ongoing.

High-Content Screening

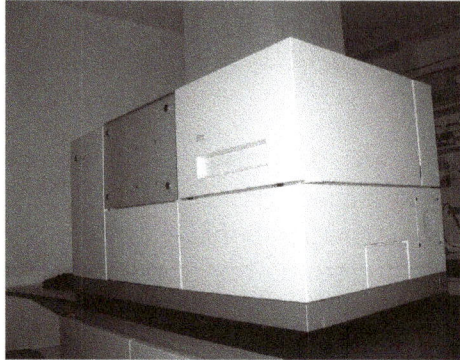

Figure: An automated confocal image reader

High throughput screens using automated imaging technology (sometimes called high-content screening) have become a standard method for both drug discovery and basic biological research. Using multi-well plates, robotics, and automated microscopy, the same assay can be applied to a large library of possible reagents (typically either small molecules or RNAi) very rapidly, obtaining thousands of images in a short amount of time. Due to the high volume of data generated, automatic image analysis is a necessity.

When positive and negative controls are available, the problem can be approached as a classification problem and the same techniques of feature computation and classification that are used for subcellular location analysis can be applied.

Segmentation

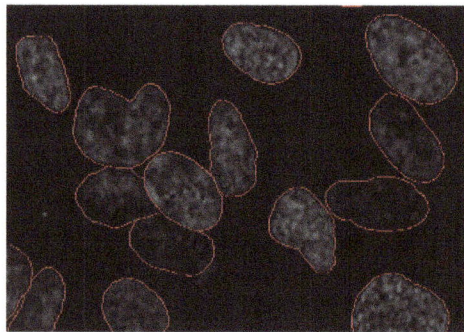

Example image for segmentation problem. Shown are nuclei of mouse NIH 3T3, stained with Hoechst and a segmentation in red.

Segmentation of cells is an important sub-problem in many of the fields below (and sometimes useful on its own if the goal is only to obtain a cell count in a viability assay). The goal is to identify the boundaries of cells in a multi-cell image. This allows for processing each cell individually to measure parameters. In 3D data, segmentation must be performed in 3D space.

As the imaging of a nuclear marker is common across many images, a widely used protocol is to segment the nuclei. This can be useful by itself if nuclear measurements are needed or it can serve to seed a watershed which extends the segmentation to the whole image.

All major segmentation methods have been reported on cell images, from simple thresholding to level set methods. Because there are multiple image modalities and different cell types, each of which implies different tradeoffs, there is no single accepted solution for this problem.

Cell image segmentation as an important procedure is often used to study gene expression and colocalization relationship etc. of individual cells. In such cases of single-cell analysis it is often needed to uniquely determine the identities of cells while segmenting the cells. Such a recognition task is often non-trivial computationally. For model organisms such as C. elegans that have well-defined cell lineages, it is possible to explicitly recognize the cell identities via image analysis, by combining both image segmentation and pattern recognition methods. Simultaneous segmentation and recognition of cells has also been proposed as a more accurate solution for this problem when an "atlas" or other prior information of cells is available. Since gene expression at single cell resolution can be obtained using these types of imaging based approaches, it is possible to combine these methods with other single cell gene expression quantification methods such as RNAseq.

Tracking

Tracking is another traditional image processing problem which appears in bioimage informatics. The problem is to relate objects that appear in subsequent frames of a film. As with segmentation, the problem can be posed in both two- and three-dimensional forms.

In the case of fluorescent imaging, tracking must often be performed on very low contrast images. As obtaining high contrast is done by shining more light which damages the sample and destroys the dye, illumination is kept at a minimum. It is often useful to think of a photon budget: the number of photons that can be used for imaging before the damage to the sample is so great that data can no longer be trusted. Therefore, if high contrast images are to be obtained, then only a few frames can be used; while for long movies, each frame will be of very low contrast.

Registration

When image data samples of different natures, such as those corresponding to different labeling methods, different individuals, samples at different time points, etc. are considered, images often need to be registered for better comparison. One example is as time-course data is collected, images in subsequent frames must often be registered so that minor shifts in the camera position can be corrected for. Another example is that when many images of a model animal (e.g. C. elegans or Drosophila brain or a mouse brain) are collected, there is often a substantial need to register these images to compare their patterns (e.g. those correspond to the same or different neuron population, those share or differ in the gene expression, etc.).

Medical image registration software packages were early attempts to be used for the microscopic image registration applications. However, due to the often much larger image file size and a much bigger number of specimens in the experiments, in many cases it is needed to develop new 3D image registration software. The BrainAligner is a software that has been used to automate the 3D deformable and nonlinear registration process using a reliable-landmark-matching strategy. It has been primarily used to generate more than 50,000 3D standardized fruitfly brain images at Janelia Farm of HHMI, with other applications including dragonfly and mice.

Important Venues

A consortium of scientists from universities and research institutes have organized annual meetings on bioimage informatics since 2005. The ISMB conference has had a *Bioimaging & Data Visualization* track since 2010. The journal Bioinformatics also introduced a *Bioimage Informatics* track in 2012. The OpenAccess journal BMC Bioinformatics has a section devoted to bioimage analysis, visualization and related applications. Other computational biology and bioinformatics journals also regularly publish bioimage informatics work.

Interactome

The interactome is the whole set of molecular interactions that occur within a particular cell. The term interactome was originally coined in 1999 by a group of French scientists headed by Bernard Jacq, and is often described in terms of biological networks. Interactomics is a discipline at the intersection of bioinformatics and biology that deals with studying both the interactions and the consequences of those interactions between and among proteins and other molecules within a cell. Molecular interactions can occur between molecules belonging to different biochemical families or within a given family, such as proteins, nucleic acids, lipids, and carbohydrates. Interactomes may be described as biological networks, and most commonly, interactome refers to protein-protein interaction (PPI) network and protein-DNA interaction networks, or subsets thereof. Therefore, a typical interactome includes transcription factors, chromatin regulatory proteins, and their target genes. Interactomics aims to compare such networks of interactions between and within species in order to discover patterns of network preservation and/or variation. Interactomic methods are currently being used to predict the function of proteins with no known function, especially in the field of drug discovery.

Experimental Methods to Map Interactomes

Network science deals with complexity by "simplifying" complex systems, summarizing them merely as components (nodes) and interactions (edges) between them. In this simplified approach, the functional richness of each node is lost. Despite or even perhaps because of such simplifications, useful discoveries can be made. As regards cellular systems, the nodes are metabolites and macromolecules such as proteins, RNA molecules and gene sequences, while the edges are physical, biochemical and functional interactions that can be identified with a plethora of technologies. One challenge of network biology is to provide maps of such interactions using systematic and standardized approaches and assays that are as unbiased as possible. The resulting "interactome" networks, the networks of interactions between cellular components, can serve as scaffold information to extract global or local graph theory properties. Once shown to be statistically different from randomized networks, such properties can then be related back to a better understanding of biological processes. Potentially powerful details of each interaction in the network are left aside, including functional, dynamic and logical features, as well as biochemical and structural aspects such as protein post-translational modifications or allosteric changes. The power of the approach resides precisely in such simplification of molecular detail, which allows modeling at the scale of whole cells.

Early attempts at experimental proteome-scale interactome network mapping in the mid-1990s were inspired by several conceptual advances in biology. The biochemistry of metabolic pathways had already given rise to cellular scale representations of metabolic networks. The discovery of signaling pathways and cross-talk between them, as well as large molecular complexes such as RNA polymerases, all involving innumerable physical protein-protein interactions, suggested the existence of highly connected webs of interactions. Finally, the rapidly growing identification of many individual interactions between transcription factors and specific DNA regulatory sequences involved in the regulation of gene expression raised the question of how transcriptional regulation is globally organized within cells.

Three distinct approaches have been used since to capture interactome networks:

i) Compilation or curation of already existing data available in the literature, usually obtained from one or just a few types of physical or biochemical interactions;

ii) Computational predictions based on available "orthogonal" information apart from physical or biochemical interactions, such as sequence similarities, gene-order conservation, co-presence and co-absence of genes in completely sequenced genomes and protein structural information; and

iii) Systematic, unbiased high-throughput experimental mapping strategies applied at the scale of whole genomes or proteomes.

These approaches, though complementary, differ greatly in the possible interpretations of the resulting maps. Literature-curated maps present the advantage of using already available information, but are limited by the inherently variable quality of the published data, the lack of systematization, and the absence of reporting of negative data. Computational prediction maps are fast and efficient to implement, and usually include satisfyingly large numbers of nodes and edges, but are necessarily imperfect because they use indirect information. While high-throughput maps attempt to describe unbiased, systematic and well-controlled data, they were initially more difficult to establish, although recent technological advances suggest that near completion can be reached within a few years for highly reliable, comprehensive protein-protein interaction and gene regulatory network maps for human.

The mapping and analysis of interactome networks for model organisms was instrumental in getting to this point. Such efforts provided, and will continue to provide, both necessary pioneering technologies and crucial conceptual insights. As with other aspects of biology, advancements in mapping of interactome networks would have been minimal without a focus on model organisms. The field of interactome mapping has been helped by developments in several model organisms, primarily the yeast *Saccharomyces cerevisiae*, the fly *Drosophila melanogaster*, and the worm *Caenorhabditis elegans*. For instance, genome-wide resources such as collections of all, or nearly all, open reading frames (ORFeomes) were first generated for these model organisms, both because their genomes are the best annotated and because there are fewer complications, such as the high number of splice variants in human and other mammals. ORFeome resources allow efficient transfer of large numbers of ORFs into vectors suitable for diverse interactome mapping technologies. Moreover, gene ablation technologies, knockouts (for yeast) and knockdowns by RNAi (for worms and flies) and transposon insertions (for plants), were discovered in and are being applied genome-wide for these model organisms.

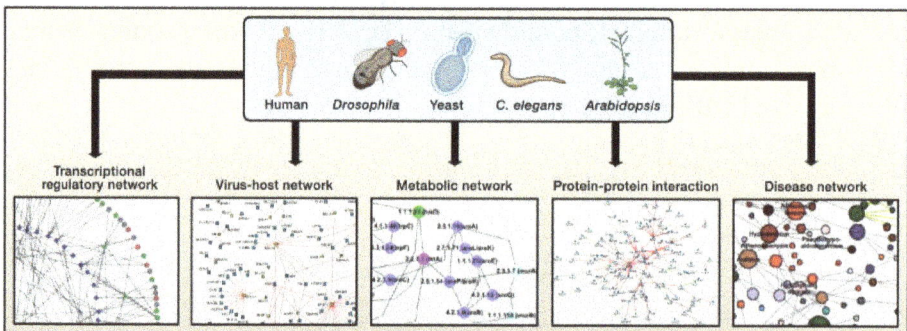

Figure : **Networks in cellular systems**

To date cellular networks are most available for the "super-model" organisms yeast, worm, fly, and plant. High-throughput interactome mapping relies upon genome-scale resources such as ORFeome resources, a segment of which is shown in the background. Several types of interactome networks discussed are depicted around the periphery. In a protein interaction network nodes represent proteins and edges represent physical interactions. In a transcriptional regulatory network nodes represent transcription factors (circular nodes) or putative DNA regulatory elements (diamond nodes) and edges represent physical binding between the two. In a gene-disease network, nodes represent disease genes and edges represent genes mutation of which is associated with disease. In a virus-host network nodes represent viral proteins (square nodes) or host proteins (round nodes) and edges represent physical interactions between the two. In a metabolic network nodes represent enzymes and edges represent metabolites that are products or substrates of the enzymes. The network depictions seem dense, but they represent only small portions of available interactome network maps, which themselves constitute only a few percent of the complete interactomes within cells.

Metabolic Networks

Metabolic network maps attempt to comprehensively describe all possible biochemical reactions for a particular cell or organism. In many representations of metabolic networks, nodes are biochemical metabolites and edges are either the reactions that convert one metabolite into another or the enzymes that catalyze these reactions. Edges can be directed or undirected, depending on whether a given reaction is reversible or not. In specific cases of metabolic network modeling, the converse situation can be used, with nodes representing enzymes and edges pointing to "adjacent" pairs of enzymes for which the product of one is the substrate of the other.

Although large metabolic pathway charts have existed for decades, nearly complete metabolic network maps required the completion of full genome sequencing together with accurate gene annotation tools. Network construction is manual with computational assistance, involving

i) The meticulous curation of large numbers of publications, each describing experimental results regarding one or several metabolic reactions characterized from purified or reconstituted enzymes, and

ii) When necessary, the compilation of predicted reactions from studies of orthologous enzymes experimentally characterized in other species.

Assembly of the union of all experimentally demonstrated and predicted reactions gives rise to proteome-scale network maps. Such maps have been compiled for numerous species, predominantly prokaryotes and unicellular eukaryotes and full-scale metabolic reconstructions are now underway for human as well. Metabolic network maps are likely the most comprehensive of all biological networks, although considerable gaps will remain to be filled in by direct experimental investigations.

Protein-Protein Interaction Networks

In protein-protein interaction network maps, nodes represent proteins and edges represent a physical interaction between two proteins. The edges are non-directed;

as it cannot be said which protein binds the other, that is, which partner functionally influences the other. Of the many methodologies that can map protein-protein interactions, two are currently in wide use for large-scale mapping. Mapping of *binary* interactions is primarily carried out by ever improving variations of the yeast two-hybrid (Y2H) system. Mapping of membership in protein complexes, providing *indirect associations* between proteins, is carried out by affinity or immuno- purification to isolate protein complexes, followed by some form of mass spectrometry (AP/MS) to identify protein constituents of these complexes. While Y2H datasets contain mostly *direct* binary interactions, AP/MS co-complex data sets are composed of direct interactions mixed with a preponderance of *indirect* associations. Accordingly, the graphs generated by these two approaches exhibit different global properties, such as the relationships between gene essentiality and the number of interacting proteins.

Computational Methods to Study Interactomes

Once an interactome has been created, there are numerous ways to analyze its properties. However, there are two important goals of such analyses. First, scientists try to elucidate the systems properties of interactomes, e.g. the topology of its interactions. Second, studies may focus on individual proteins and their role in the network. Such analyses are mainly carried out using bioinformatics methods and include the following, among many others:

Validation

First, the coverage and quality of an interactome has to be evaluated. Interactomes are never complete, given the limitations of experimental methods. For instance, it has been estimated that typical Y2H screens detect only 25% or so of all interactions in an interactome. The coverage of an interactome can be assessed by comparing it to benchmarks of well-known interactions that have been found and validated by independent assays. Other methods filter out false positives calculating the similarity of known annotations of the proteins involved or define a likelihood of interaction using the subcellular localization of these proteins.

Predicting PPIs

Using experimental data as a starting point, *homology transfer* is one way to predict interactomes. Here, PPIs from one organism are used to predict interactions among homologous proteins in another organism. However, this approach has certain limitations, primarily because the source data may not be reliable (e.g. contain false positives and false negatives). In addition, proteins and their interactions change during evolution and thus may have been lost or gained. Nevertheless, numerous interactomes have been predicted, e.g. that of *Bacillus licheniformis*.

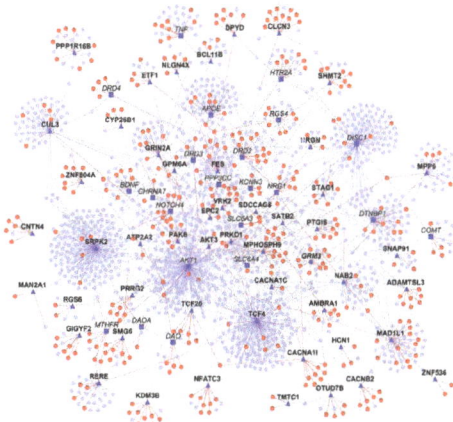

Schziophrenia PPI.

Some algorithms use experimental evidence on structural complexes, the atomic details of binding interfaces and produce detailed atomic models of protein–protein complexes as well as other protein–molecule interactions. Other algorithms use only sequence information, thereby creating unbiased complete networks of interaction with many mistakes.

Some methods use machine learning to distinguish how interacting protein pairs differ from non-interacting protein pairs in terms of pairwise features such as cellular colocalization, gene co-expression, how closely located on a DNA are the genes that encode the two proteins, and so on. Random Forest has been found to be most-effective machine learning method for protein interaction prediction. Such methods have been applied for discovering protein interactions on human interactome, specifically the interactome of Membrane proteins and the interactome of Schizophrenia-associated proteins.

Text Mining of PPIs

Some efforts have been made to extract systematically interaction networks directly from the scientific literature. Such approaches range in terms of complexity from simple co-occurrence statistics of entities that are mentioned together in the same context (e.g. sentence) to sophisticated natural language processing and machine learning methods for detecting interaction relationships.

Protein Function Prediction

Protein interaction networks have been used to predict the function of proteins of unknown functions. This is usually based on the assumption that uncharacterized proteins have similar functions as their interacting proteins. For example, YbeB, a protein of unknown function was found to interact with ribosomal proteins and later shown to be involved in translation. Although such predictions may be based on single interactions, usually several interactions are found. Thus, the whole network of interactions can be used to predict protein functions, given that certain functions are usually enriched among the interactors.

Perturbations and Disease

The *topology* of an interactome makes certain predictions how a network reacts to the perturbation (e.g. removal) of nodes (proteins) or edges (interactions). Such perturbations can be caused by mutations of genes, and thus their proteins and a network reaction can manifest as a disease. A network analysis can identify drug targets and biomarkers of diseases.

Network Structure and Topology

Interaction networks can be analyzed using the tools of graph theory. Network properties include the degree distribution, clustering coefficients, betweenness centrality, and many others. The distribution of properties among the proteins of an interactome has revealed that the interactome networks often have scale-free topology where functional modules within a network indicate specialized subnetworks. Such modules can be functional, as in a signaling pathway, or structural, as in a protein complex. In fact, it is a formidable task to identify protein complexes in an interactome, given that a network on its own does not directly reveal the presence of a stable complex.

Network Properties

Protein interaction networks can be analyzed with the same tool as other networks. In fact, they share many properties with biological or social networks. Some of the main characteristics are as follows.

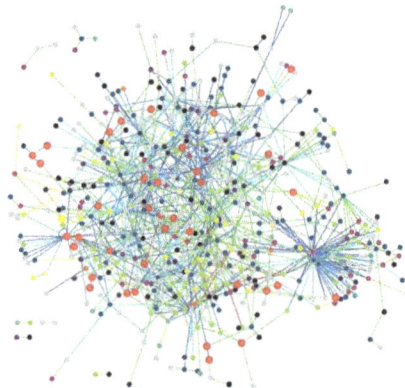

Figure: The *Treponema pallidum* protein interactome.

Degree Distribution

The degree distribution describes the number of proteins that have a certain number of connections. Most protein interaction networks show a scale-free (power law) degree distribution where the connectivity distribution $P(k) \sim k^{-\gamma}$ with k being the degree. This relationship can also be seen as a straight line on a log-log plot since, the above equation is equal to $\log(P(k)) \sim -\gamma \cdot \log(k)$. One characteristic of such distributions is that there are many proteins with few interactions and few proteins that have many interactions, the latter being called "hubs".

Hubs

Highly connected nodes (proteins) are called hubs. Han et al. have coined the term "party hub" for hubs whose expression is correlated with its interaction partners. Party hubs also connect proteins within functional modules such as protein complexes. In contrast, "date hubs" do not exhibit such a correlation and appear to connect different functional modules. Party hubs are found predominantly in AP/MS data sets, whereas date hubs are found predominantly in binary interactome network maps. Note that the validity of the date hub/party hub distinction was disputed. Party hubs generally consist of multi-interface proteins whereas date hubs are more frequently single-interaction interface proteins. Consistent with a role for date-hubs in connecting different processes, in yeast the number of binary interactions of a given protein is correlated to the number of phenotypes observed for the corresponding mutant gene in different physiological conditions.

Modules

Nodes involved in the same biochemical process are highly interconnected.

Flow Cytometry Bioinformatics

Flow cytometry (FCM) is a technology that is commonly used for the rapid characterization of cells of the immune system at the single cell level based on antigens presented on the cell surface. Cells of interest are targeted by a set of fluorochrome-conjugated antibodies (markers) and pass through a laser beam one-by-one at over 10 000 cells per minute. Scattered light of different wavelengths for each marker is measured and recorded by sensitive detectors. This subsequently creates a unique intensity profile that allows for differentiation of cell types. FCM is widely used in research, for example in immunophenotyping where it holds great promise for assessing the immune status of patient populations. Within a blood or tissue sample, the most common measurement of interest is cell frequency (i.e. the proportion of a cell population), either absolute or relative to a parent population. Variations in cell frequencies can give important information about the immune status or allow association of cell types with a biological variable.

The accurate determination of cell population frequencies is a key aim in FCM analysis. Using differential expression of one or more markers, it is possible to delineate cell populations of interest, a process commonly known as 'gating'. This task usually comprises the manual inspection of bivariate density plots using marker channels that were selected from prior biological knowledge. Subsequently, for each sample, cell populations are identified by drawing regions of interest or setting channel thresholds. While some populations are easy to gate, populations with very small cell proportions (rare populations) can be challenging. Large populations can obscure rare ones, such that they do not necessarily appear as clusters or well pronounced density peaks, hence are difficult to detect. Due to the large number of possible combinations of markers, gating is a labor intensive and highly subjective process. In contrast, automated methods offer little to no bias and comparable variability. Thus, there has been substantial interest in developing methods that ease the process of identifying cell populations as much as possible, and a large variety of tools, both unsupervised and supervised, have been developed.

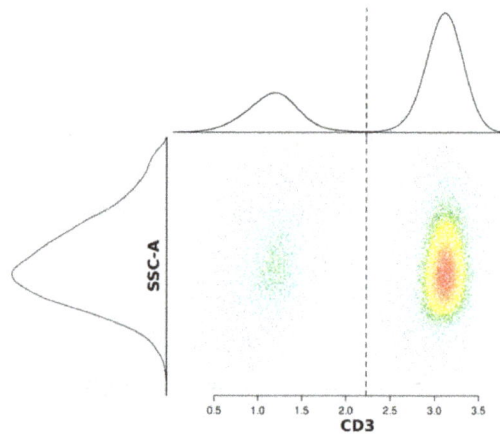

Figure: Density plot for two channels 'CD-3' against 'SSC-A'. Each dot represents a cell and corresponding one-dimensional densities are attached at the top and left.

The shown data is an example of gating T-cells from lymphocyte singlet cells. Axis values correspond to intensity values. Knowing that T-cells (right cluster) express CD3, they can be delineated from other lymphocytes (left cluster). The corresponding density estimates for both channels are shown along the left and top axis. The CD3 threshold is located in a valley between the density peaks from both populations

Several tools are based on sophisticated techniques from machine learning, i.e. dimensionality reduction, clustering and deep learning. They aim to eliminate the traditional approach of inspecting bivariate channels plots by considering all channels at once instead of only two at a time. While these methods have shown very good performance on many datasets, they still suffer from a few major drawbacks, especially pronounced for large sets of highly diverse FCM samples. First, in high-dimensional spaces, cells do not necessarily form distinct clusters that would be easily discoverable. It is visible that both child populations are not distinct from each other. Consequently, for an approach solely based on this technology, it is highly difficult to gate both complex populations. Second, in order to describe populations of interest, the

fine-tuning of a set of hyper-parameters is crucial and common to all tools, in particular in the context of small populations where the underlying machine learning task is
quite challenging. Hyper-parameters are values controlling the result of an automated method, typically set by practitioners in a way that the outcome of the method is
satisfactory. Often, hyper-parameters do not have an intuitive meaning, but relate to
mathematical or algorithmic characteristics of the method. Depending on the method, practitioners might not have the required knowledge to set those optimally. In the
presence of high sample diversity, fine-tuning such parameters is essential and might
take a significant amount of time. Due to the difficulties in finding an optimal set of
parameters, it is also complicated to compare such tools. Third, when incorporating
machine learning, interpretability of results is limited, leading to a lack of general
understanding of how such methods work. Hence, it is problematic to verify gates
from a biological standpoint.

In FCM studies, quality checking of results is an essential step in the accurate identification of populations, and ensures that no wrong conclusions are drawn from the data
in later steps. For that reason, and also because of the familiarity with the traditional
approach of inspecting bivariate density plots, for quality checking, manual gating is
the current standard practice.

FlowDensity takes another point of view and tries to automate the threshold selection based on density shape features. The algorithm can work in both an unsupervised
or supervised fashion. When customizing thresholds on a per-population level, one or
more channels are inspected, and density features such as differences in extrema, slope
changes, or the numbers of peaks are examined, generally based on a pre-determined
manual gating hierarchy. Gates in the form of channel thresholds are estimated, from
which sub-populations can be extracted. Provided hyper-parameters are appropriately
chosen, flow. Density offers a state-of-the-art tool for the accurate identification of cell
populations that matches what would have been obtained through manual analysis.
Once the rules for each population are set, thresholds are automatically and individually set for each new data file, similar to the manual tweaking that operators tend to do,
but in a data-driven fashion. As a result, flowDensity results are robust, reproducible
and the approach performs better than the manual alternative it is designed to match.
However, undertaking a supervised setup does require a significant time component in
order to obtain the optimal results.

Data Collection

Flow cytometers operate by hydrodynamically focusing suspended cells so that they
separate from each other within a fluid stream. The stream is interrogated by one or
more lasers, and the resulting fluorescent and scattered light is detected by photomul-
tipliers. By using optical filters, particular fluorophores on or within the cells can be
quantified by peaks in their emission spectra. These may be endogenous fluorophores
such as chlorophyll or transgenic green fluorescent protein, or they may be artificial

fluorophores covalently bonded to detection molecules such as antibodies for detecting proteins, or hybridization probes for detecting DNA or RNA.

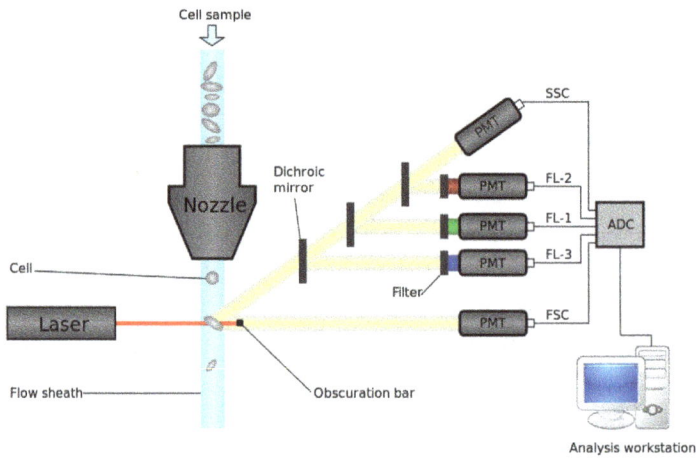

Figure: Schematic diagram of a flow cytometer, showing focusing of the fluid sheath, laser, optics, photomultiplier tubes, analogue-to-digital converter, and analysis workstation

The ability to quantify these has led to flow cytometry being used in a wide range of applications, including but not limited to:

- Monitoring of CD4 count in HIV.

- Diagnosis of various cancers.

- Analysis of aquatic microbiomes.

- Sperm sorting.

- Measuring telomere length.

Until the early 2000s, flow cytometry could only measure a few fluorescent markers at a time. Through the late 1990s into the mid-2000s, however, rapid development of new fluorophores resulted in modern instruments capable of quantifying up to 18 markers per cell. More recently, the new technology of mass cytometry replaces fluorophores with rare-earth elements detected by time of flight mass spectrometry, achieving the ability to measure the expression of 34 or more markers. At the same time, microfluidic qPCR methods are providing a flow cytometry-like method of quantifying 48 or more RNA molecules per cell. The rapid increase in the dimensionality of flow cytometry data, coupled with the development of high-throughput robotic platforms capable of assaying hundreds to thousands of samples automatically have created a need for improved computational analysis methods.

Data

Flow cytometry data is in the form of a large matrix of intensities over M wavelengths by N events. Most events will be a particular cell, although some may be doublets (pairs of cells which pass the laser closely together). For each event, the measured fluorescence intensity over a particular wavelength range is recorded.

Markers

Figure: Representation of flow cytometry data from an instrument with three scatters channels and 13 fluorescent channels. Only the values for the first 30 (of hundreds of thousands) of cells are shown.

The measured fluorescence intensity indicates the amount of that fluorophore in the cell, which indicates the amount that has bound to detector molecules such as antibodies. Therefore, fluorescence intensity can be considered a proxy for the amount of detector molecules present on the cell. A simplified, if not strictly accurate, way of considering flow cytometry data is as a matrix of M measurements of amounts of molecules of interest by N cells.

Steps in Computational Flow Cytometry Data Analysis

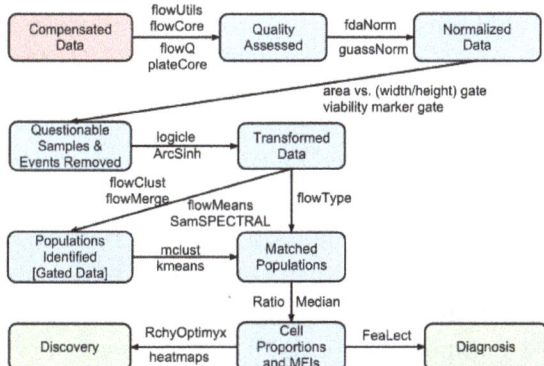

Figure: An example pipeline for analysis of FCM data and some of the Bioconductor packages relevant to each step.

The process of moving from primary FCM data to disease diagnosis and biomarker discovery involves four major steps:

1. Data pre-processing (including compensation, transformation and normalization).

2. Cell population identification (a.k.a. gating).

3. Cell population matching for cross sample comparison.

4. Relating cell populations to external variables (diagnosis and discovery).

Saving of the steps taken in a particular flow cytometry workflow is supported by some flow cytometry software, and is important for the reproducibility of flow cytometry experiments. However, saved workspace files are rarely interchangeable between software. An attempt to solve this problem is the development of the Gating-ML XML-based data standard (discussed in more detail under the standards section), which is slowly being adopted in both commercial and open source flow cytometry software. The CytoML R package is also filling the gap by importing/exporting the Gating-ML that is compatible with FlowJo, CytoBank and FACS Diva softwares.

Data Pre-processing

Prior to analysis, flow cytometry data must typically undergo pre-processing to remove artifacts and poor quality data, and to be transformed onto an optimal scale for identifying cell populations of interest. Below are various steps in a typical flow cytometry preprocessing pipeline.

Compensation

When more than one fluorochrome is used with the same laser, their emission spectra frequently overlap. Each particular fluorochrome is typically measured using a bandpass optical filter set to a narrow band at or near the fluorochrome's emission intensity peak. The result is that the reading for any given fluorochrome is actually the sum of that fluorochrome's peak emission intensity, and the intensity of all other fluorochromes' spectra where they overlap with that frequency band. This overlap is termed spillover, and the process of removing spillover from flow cytometry data is called compensation.

Compensation is typically accomplished by running a series of representative samples each stained for only one fluorochrome, to give measurements of the contribution of each fluorochrome to each channel. The total signal to remove from each channel can be computed by solving a system of linear equations based on this data to produce a spillover matrix, which when inverted and multiplied with the raw data from the cytometer produces the compensated data. The processes of computing the spillover matrix, or applying a precomputed spillover matrix to compensate flow cytometry data, are standard features of flow cytometry software.

Transformation

Cell populations detected by flow cytometry are often described as having approximately log-normal expression. As such, they have traditionally been transformed to a logarithmic scale. In early cytometers, this was often accomplished even before data acquisition by use of a log amplifier. On modern instruments, data is usually stored in linear form, and transformed digitally prior to analysis.

However, compensated flow cytometry data frequently contains negative values due to compensation, and cell populations do occur which have low means and normal distributions. Logarithmic transformations cannot properly handle negative values, and poorly display normally distributed cell types. Alternative transformations which address this issue include the log-linear hybrid transformations Logicle and Hyperlog, as well as the hyperbolic arcsine and the Box-Cox.

A comparison of commonly used transformations concluded that the biexponential and Box-Cox transformations, when optimally parameterized, provided the clearest visualization and least variance of cell populations across samples. However, a later comparison of the flow Trans package used in that comparison indicated that it did not parameterize the Logicle transformation in a manner consistent with other implementations, potentially calling those results into question.

Quality Control

Particularly in newer, high-throughput experiments, there is a need for visualization methods to help detect technical errors in individual samples. One approach is to visualize summary statistics, such as the empirical distribution functions of single dimensions of technical or biological replicates to ensure they are the similar. For more rigor, the Kolmogorov–Smirnov test can be used to determine if individual samples deviate from the norm. The Grubbs' test for outliers may be used to detect samples deviating from the group.

A method for quality control in higher-dimensional space is to use probability binning with bins fit to the whole data set pooled together. Then the standard deviation of the number of cells falling in the bins within each sample can be taken as a measure of multidimensional similarity, with samples that are closer to the norm having a smaller standard deviation. With this method, higher standard deviation can indicate outliers, although this is a relative measure as the absolute value depends partly on the number of bins.

With all of these methods, the cross-sample variation is being measured. However, this is the combination of technical variations introduced by the instruments and handling, and actual biological information that is desired to be measured. Disambiguating the technical and the biological contributions to between-sample variation can be a difficult to impossible task.

Normalization

Particularly in multi-center studies, technical variation can make biologically equivalent populations of cells difficult to match across samples. Normalization methods to remove technical variance, frequently derived from image registration techniques, are thus a critical step in many flow cytometry analyses. Single-marker normalization can be performed using landmark registration, in which peaks in a kernel density estimate of each sample are identified and aligned across samples.

Identifying Cell Populations

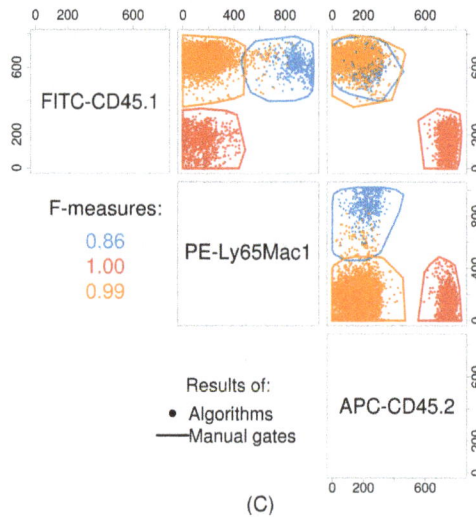

(C)

Two-dimensional scatter plots covering all three combinations of three chosen dimensions. The colors show the comparison of consensus of eight independent manual gates (polygons) and automated gates (colored dots). The consensus of the manual gates and the algorithms were produced using the CLUE package. Figure reproduced from.

The complexity of raw flow cytometry data (dozens of measurements for thousands to millions of cells) makes answering questions directly using statistical tests or supervised learning difficult. Thus, a critical step in the analysis of flow cytometric data is to reduce this complexity to something more tractable while establishing common features across samples. This usually involves identifying multidimensional regions that contain functionally and phenotypically homogeneous groups of cells. This is a form of cluster analysis. There are a range of methods by which this can be achieved, detailed below.

Gating

The data generated by flow-cytometers can be plotted in one or two dimensions to produce a histogram or scatter plot. The regions on these plots can be sequentially separated, based on fluorescence intensity, by creating a series of subset extractions, termed "gates". These gates can be produced using software, e.g. Flowjo, FCS Express, WinMDI, CytoPaint (aka Paint-A-Gate), VenturiOne, Cellcion, CellQuest Pro, Cytospec, Kaluza. or flowCore.

In datasets with a low number of dimensions and limited cross-sample technical and biological variability (e.g., clinical laboratories), manual analysis of specific cell populations can produce effective and reproducible results. However, exploratory analysis of a large number of cell populations in a high-dimensional dataset is not feasible. In addition, manual analysis in less controlled settings (e.g., cross-laboratory studies) can increase the overall error rate of the study. In one study, several computational gating algorithms performed better than manual analysis in the presence of some variation. However, despite the considerable advances in computational analysis, manual gating remains the main solution for the identification of specific rare cell populations that are not well-separated from other cell types.

Gating Guided by Dimension Reduction

The number of scatter plots that need to be investigated increases with the square of the number of markers measured (or faster since some markers need to be investigated several times for each group of cells to resolve high-dimensional differences between cell types that appear to be similar in most markers). To address this issue, principal component analysis has been used to summarize the high-dimensional datasets using a combination of markers that maximizes the variance of all data points. However, PCA is a linear method and is not able to preserve complex and non-linear relationships. More recently, two dimensional minimum spanning tree layouts have been used to guide the manual gating process. Density-based down-sampling and clustering was used to better represent rare populations and control the time and memory complexity of the minimum spanning tree construction process. More sophisticated dimension reduction algorithms are yet to be investigated.

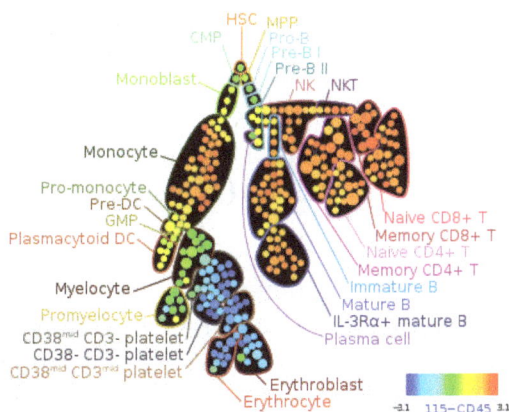

Figure: Cell populations in a high-dimensional mass-cytometry dataset manually gated after dimension reduction using 2D layout for a minimum spanning tree. Figure reproduced from the data provided in.

Automated Gating

Developing computational tools for identification of cell populations has been an area of active research only since 2008. Many individual clustering approaches have recently been developed, including model-based algorithms (e.g., flowClust and FLAME), density based algorithms (e.g. FLOCK and SWIFT, graph-based approaches (e.g. Sam-SPECTRAL) and most recently, hybrids of several approaches (flowMeans and flow-Peaks). These algorithms are different in terms of memory and time complexity, their software requirements, their ability to automatically determine the required number of cell populations, and their sensitivity and specificity. The FlowCAP (Flow Cytometry: Critical Assessment of Population Identification Methods) project, with active participation from most academic groups with research efforts in the area, is providing a way to objectively cross-compare state-of-the-art automated analysis approaches. Other surveys have also compared automated gating tools on several datasets.

Probability Binning Methods

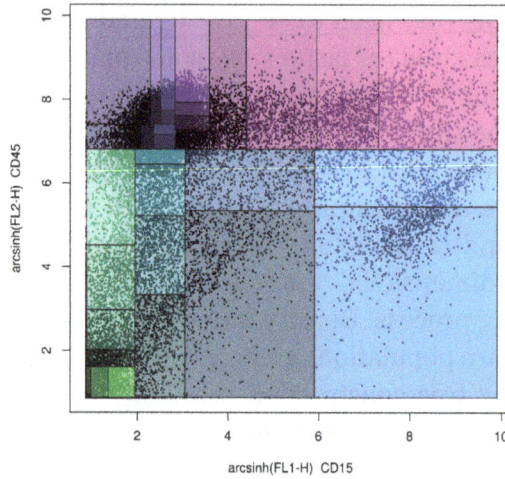

Figure: An example of frequency difference gating, created using the flowFP Bioconductor package. The dots represent individual events in an FCS file. The rectangles represent the bins.

Probability binning is a non-gating analysis method in which flow cytometry data is split into quantiles on a univariate basis. The locations of the quantiles can then be used to test for differences between samples (in the variables not being split) using the chi-squared test.

This was later extended into multiple dimensions in the form of frequency difference gating, a binary space partitioning technique where data is iteratively partitioned along the median. These partitions (or bins) are fit to a control sample. Then the proportion of cells falling within each bin in test samples can be compared to the control sample by the chi squared test.

Finally, cytometric fingerprinting uses a variant of frequency difference gating to set bins and measure for a series of samples how many cells fall within each bin. These bins can be used as gates and used for subsequent analysis similarly to automated gating methods.

Combinatorial Gating

High-dimensional clustering algorithms are often unable to identify rare cell types that are not well separated from other major populations. Matching these small cell populations across multiple samples is even more challenging. In manual analysis, prior biological knowledge (e.g., biological controls) provides guidance to reasonably identify these populations. However, integrating this information into the exploratory clustering process (e.g., as in semi-supervised learning) has not been successful.

An alternative to high-dimensional clustering is to identify cell populations using one marker at a time and then combine them to produce higher-dimensional clusters. This functionality was first implemented in FlowJo. The flowType algorithm builds on this framework by allowing the exclusion of the markers. This enables the development of statistical tools (e.g. RchyOptimyx) that can investigate the importance of each marker and exclude high-dimensional redundancies.

Diagnosis and Discovery

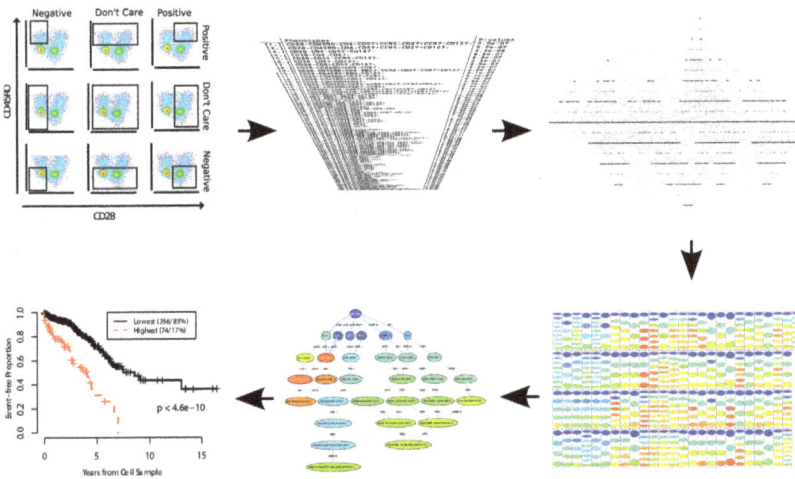

Figure: Overview of the flowType/RchyOptimyx pipeline for identification of correlates of protection against HIV:

First, tens of thousands of cell populations are identified by combining one-dimensional partitions (panel one). The cell populations are then analyzed using a statistical test (and bonferroni's method for multiple testing correction) to identify those correlated with the survival information. The third panel shows a complete gating hierarchy describing all possible strategies for gating that cell population. This graph can be mined to identify the "best" gating strategy (i.e., the one in which the most important markers appear earlier). These hierarchies for all selected phenotypes are demonstrated in panel 4. In panel 5, these hierarchies are merged into a single graph that summarized the entire dataset and demonstrates the trade-off between the number of markers involved in each phenotype and the significance of the correlation with the clinical outcome.

After identification of the cell population of interest, a cross sample analysis can be performed to identify phenotypical or functional variations that are correlated with an external variable (e.g., a clinical outcome). These studies can be partitioned into two main groups:

Diagnosis

In these studies, the goal usually is to diagnose a disease (or a sub-class of a disease) using variations in one or more cell populations. For example, one can use multidimensional clustering to identify a set of clusters, match them across all samples, and then use supervised learning to construct a classifier for prediction of the classes of interest (e.g., this approach can be used to improve the accuracy of the classification of specific lymphoma subtypes). Alternatively, all the cells from the entire cohort can be pooled into a single multidimensional space for clustering before classification. This approach is particularly suitable for datasets with a high amount of biological variation (in which cross-sample matching is challenging) but requires technical variations to be carefully controlled.

Discovery

In a discovery setting, the goal is to identify and describe cell populations correlated with an external variable (as opposed to the diagnosis setting in which the goal is to combine the predictive power of multiple cell types to maximize the accuracy of the results). Similar to the diagnosis use-case, cluster matching in high-dimensional space can be used for exploratory analysis but the descriptive power of this approach is very limited, as it is hard to characterize and visualize a cell population in a high-dimensional space without first reducing the dimensionality. Finally, combinatorial gating approaches have been particularly successful in exploratory analysis of FCM data. Simplified Presentation of Incredibly Complex Evaluations (SPICE) is a software package that can use the gating functionality of FlowJo to statistically evaluate a wide range of different cell populations and visualize those that are correlated with the external outcome. flowType and RchyOptimyx expand this technique by adding the ability of exploring the impact of independent markers on the overall correlation with the external outcome. This enables the removal of unnecessary markers and provides a simple visualization of all identified cell types. In a recent analysis of a large (n=466) cohort of HIV+ patients, this pipeline identified three correlates of protection against HIV, only one of which had been previously identified through extensive manual analysis of the same dataset.

Data Formats and Interchange

Flow Cytometry Standard

Flow Cytometry Standard (FCS) was developed in 1984 to allow recording and sharing of flow cytometry data. Since then, FCS became the standard file format supported by all flow cytometry software and hardware vendors. The FCS specification has traditionally been developed and maintained by the International Society for Advancement of Cytometry (ISAC). Over the years, updates were incorporated to adapt to technological advancements in both flow cytometry and computing technologies with FCS

2.0 introduced in 1990, FCS 3.0 in 1997, and the most current specification FCS 3.1 in 2010. FCS used to be the only widely adopted file format in flow cytometry. Recently, additional standard file formats have been developed by ISAC.

netCDF

ISAC is considering replacing FCS with a flow cytometry specific version of the Network Common Data Form (netCDF) file format. netCDF is a set of freely available software libraries and machine independent data formats that support the creation, access, and sharing of array-oriented scientific data. In 2008, ISAC drafted the first version of netCDF conventions for storage of raw flow cytometry data.

Archival Cytometry Standard (ACS)

The Archival Cytometry Standard (ACS) is being developed to bundle data with different components describing cytometry experiments. It captures relations among data, metadata, analysis files and other components, and includes support for audit trails, versioning and digital signatures. The ACS container is based on the ZIP file format with an XML-based table of contents specifying relations among files in the container. The XML Signature W3C Recommendation has been adopted to allow for digital signatures of components within the ACS container. An initial draft of ACS has been designed in 2007 and finalized in 2010. Since then, ACS support has been introduced in several software tools including FlowJo and Cytobank.

Gating-ML

The lack of gating interoperability has traditionally been a bottleneck preventing reproducibility of flow cytometry data analysis and the usage of multiple analytical tools. To address this shortcoming, ISAC developed Gating-ML, an XML-based mechanism to formally describe gates and related data (scale) transformations. The draft recommendation version of Gating-ML was approved by ISAC in 2008 and it is partially supported by tools like FlowJo, the flowUtils, CytoML libraries in R/BioConductor, and FlowRepository. It supports rectangular gates, polygon gates, convex polytopes, ellipsoids, decision trees and Boolean collections of any of the other types of gates. In addition, it includes dozens of built in public transformations that have been shown to potentially useful for display or analysis of cytometry data. In 2013, Gating-ML version 2.0 was approved by ISAC's Data Standards Task Force as a Recommendation. This new version offers slightly less flexibility in terms of the power of gating description; however, it is also significantly easier to implement in software tools.

Classification Results (CLR)

The Classification Results (CLR) File Format has been developed to exchange the results of manual gating and algorithmic classification approaches in a standard way in order to be able to report and process the classification. CLR is based in the commonly supported CSV file format with columns corresponding to different classes and cell values containing the probability of an event being a member of a particular class. These are captured as values between 0 and 1. Simplicity of the format and its compatibility with common spreadsheet tools have been the major requirements driving the design of the specification. Although it was originally designed for the field of flow cytometry, it is applicable in any domain that needs to capture either fuzzy or unambiguous classifications of virtually any kinds of objects.

Public Data and Software

As in other bioinformatics fields, development of new methods has primarily taken the form of free open source software, and several databases have been created for depositing open data.

Bioconductor

The Bioconductor project is a repository of free open source software, mostly written in the R programming language. As of July 2013, Bioconductor contained 21 software packages for processing flow cytometry data. These packages cover most of the range of functionality described earlier in this article.

Gene Pattern

Gene Pattern is a predominantly genomic analysis platform with over 200 tools for analysis of gene expression, proteomics, and other data. A web-based interface provides easy access to these tools and allows the creation of automated analysis pipelines enabling reproducible research. Recently, a GenePattern Flow Cytometry Suite has been developed in order to bring advanced flow cytometry data analysis tools to experimentalists without programmatic skills. It contains close to 40 open source GenePattern flow cytometry modules covering methods from basic processing of flow cytometry standard (i.e., FCS) files to advanced algorithms for automated identification of cell populations, normalization and quality assessment. Internally, most of these modules leverage functionality developed in BioConductor.

Much of the functionality of the Bioconductor packages for flow cytometry analysis has been packaged up for use with the GenePattern workflow system, in the form of the GenePattern Flow Cytometry Suite.

FACSanadu

FACSanadu is an open source portable application for visualization and analysis of FCS data. Unlike Bioconductor, it is an interactive program aimed at non-programmers for routine analysis. It supports standard FCS files as well as COPAS profile data.

Public Databases

The Minimum Information about a Flow Cytometry Experiment (MIFlowCyt), requires that any flow cytometry data used in a publication be available, although this does not include a requirement that it be deposited in a public database. Thus, although the journals Cytometry Part A and B, as well as all journals from the Nature Publishing Group require MIFlowCyt compliance, there is still relatively little publicly available flow cytometry data. Some efforts have been made towards creating public databases, however.

Firstly, CytoBank, which is a complete web-based flow cytometry data storage and analysis platform, has been made available to the public in a limited form. Using the CytoBank code base, FlowRepository was developed in 2012 with the support of ISAC to be a public repository of flow cytometry data. FlowRepository facilitates MIFlowCyt compliance, and as of July 2013 contained 65 public data sets.

Datasets

In 2012, the flow cytometry community has started to release a set of publicly available datasets. A subset of these datasets representing the existing data analysis challenges is described below. For comparison against manual gating, the FlowCAP-I project has released five datasets, manually gated by human analysts, and two of them gated by eight independent analysts. The FlowCAP-II project included three datasets for binary classification and also reported several algorithms that were able to classify these samples perfectly. FlowCAP-III included two larger datasets for comparison against manual gates as well as one more challenging sample classification dataset. As of March 2013, public release of FlowCAP-III was still in progress. The datasets used in FlowCAP-I, II, and III either have a low number of subjects or parameters. However, recently several more complex clinical datasets have been released including a dataset of 466 HIV-infected subjects, which provides both 14 parameter assays and sufficient clinical information for survival analysis.

Another class of datasets is higher-dimensional mass cytometry assays. A representative of this class of datasets is a study which includes analysis of two bone marrow samples using more than 30 surface or intracellular markers under a wide range of different stimulations. The raw data for this dataset is publicly available as described in the manuscript, and manual analyses of the surface markers are available upon request from the authors.

Biodiversity Informatics

Biodiversity informatics is the application of informatics techniques to biodiversity data, is rooted in physical objects and nomenclatural codes.

The Convention on Biological Diversity (CBD) has three main objectives:

1. Conservation of Biological Diversity.

2. Sustainable use of its resources.

3. Fair and equitable share of the genetic and other resources of biological diversity.

Since biodiversity conservation is a multidisciplinary science, it seeks help and applies the principles of many other disciplines such as ecology, taxonomy, systematics, biogeography, geoinformatics, molecular biology, population genetics, philosophy, anthropology, sociology, information technology, economics etc. For conservation biologists or biodiversity experts it is a challenge to preserve the evolutionary potential and ecological viability of a vast array of biodiversity, and preserve the complex nature, dynamics and interrelationships of natural systems.

Need for Biodiversity Informatics

Much of the biodiversity information is available in the form of scientific collections such as specimens, herbaria, microorganism repositories in various universities, natural history museums, research institutions and organizations concentrated mainly in developed countries. Experts are often asked for quick advice or input by government and private agencies regarding issues such as status of a species population in a particular region or area, potential effects of introduced species, forest fire impacts in a protected area, ecological effects of development, and so on. Such experts are often hamstrung by the lack of easily accessible information.

Therefore, the need of the hour is to digitize all the available information on biodiversity and place it on information networks to aid the current generation of researchers.

Many international conservation information networks have been developed during the last few decades (see Table), most of which are open to public. These information networks include news, expertise, searchable databases, and any other kind of relevant material that can be put on websites.

Some major databases providing online information services for conservation		
Name	Website	Description
GBIF	https://www.gbif.org/ Hotspots	Global biodiversity facility, unit level records
Hotspots	https://www.conservation.org/How/Pages/Hotspots.	Provides information on global hotspots
ETI-WBD	http://www.eti.uva.nl/tools/wbd.php	Global taxonomic database
IUCN SIS	https://www.iucn.org/themes/ssc/our_work/sis.htm	IUCN Information service on species

IUCN Redlist	http://www.iucnredlist.org	IUCN information on conservation status of species
UNEP-WCMC	https://www.unep-wcmc.org	Information centre with multiple databases on conservation

The databases are playing an important role in providing baseline as well as key information to many scientists and researchers working for conservation projects in different regions of the world. They have also inspired others to develop databases and information networks for ease of information dissemination and networking in their area of expertise.

The information networks may be regional or global and may be complex or fairly simple in structure depending upon their objectives. Nevertheless, experts involved in constructing these information networks tend to make them user-friendly for public convenience.

At the global level, GBIF is playing a lead role and is the most ambitious of all information networks as far as integration of biodiversity data is concerned. GBIF's data portal is already available online as a standard source providing integrated primary data (label or observational) on all species of living organisms. It does this by providing software and web services (using extensible markup language, or XML) that enable integration of data drawn from multiple resources distributed around the world.

GBIF is currently serving over 10 million records from 34 distributed databases and intends to make the entire world's biodiversity information available to all within the next 10 year period. The GBIF mission statement is "to make the world's primary data on biodiversity freely and universally available via the Internet". Currently, 47 countries and 32 international organizations are members in GBIF, and the membership steadily grows, as does the data content. Ocean Biogeographic Information System (OBIS) is among the largest data providers to the GBIF.

Benefits of Biodiversity Informatics

- Permits mining, capture, storage, search, retrieval, visualization, mapping, modeling, analysis and publication of data.

- Networking of databases between different institutions, laboratories, universities, and research organizations that will help scientists and research scholars carry out research on different aspects of biodiversity conservation.

- Access to useful data at little or no cost with interactive and user defined readability.

- Improved education and training process as teachers can obtain real data sets for various student exercises.

- Improved education and training process as teachers can obtain real data sets for various student exercises.

- Information and data gaps are more apparent, and these gaps will encourage scientists to carry out research on the neglected, unexplored and much awaited themes and issues.

- Increased public confidence and participation in more transparent and accessible science.

References

- Wong, K. C. (2016). Computational Biology and Bioinformatics: Gene Regulation. CRC Press/ Taylor & Francis Group. ISBN 9781498724975

- Hogeweg P (1978). "Simulating the growth of cellular forms". Simulation. 31 (3): 90– 96. doi:10.1177/003754977803100305

- Bioinformatics, science: britannica.com, Retrieved 30 June 2018

- Attwood TK, Gisel A, Eriksson NE, Bongcam-Rudloff E (2011). "Concepts, Historical Milestones and the Central Place of Bioinformatics in Modern Biology: A European Perspective". Bioinformatics – Trends and Methodologies. InTech. Retrieved 8 Jan 2012

- Hoy, JA; Robinson, H; Trent JT, 3rd; Kakar, S; Smagghe, BJ; Hargrove, MS (3 August 2007). "Plant hemoglobins: a molecular fossil record for the evolution of oxygen transport". Journal of Molecular Biology. 371 (1): 168–79. doi:10.1016/j.jmb.2007.05.029. PMID 17560601

- Introduction-to-Structural-Bioinformatics-268231263: researchgate.net, Retrieved 12 July 2018

- Moody, Glyn (2004). Digital Code of Life: How Bioinformatics is Revolutionizing Science, Medicine, and Business. ISBN 978-0-471-32788-2

- Eck RV, Dayhoff MO (1966). "Evolution of the structure of ferredoxin based on living relics of primitive amino Acid sequences". Science. 152 (3720): 363–6. Bibcode:1966Sci...152..363E. doi:10.1126/science.152.3720.363. PMID 17775169

- Interactome, biochemistry-genetics-and-molecular-biology: sciencedirect.com, Retrieved 29 May 2018

- Brohée, Sylvain; Barriot, Roland; Moreau, Yves. "Biological knowledge bases using Wikis: combining the flexibility of Wikis with the structure of databases". Bioinformatics. Oxford Journals. Retrieved 5 May 2015

- Shariff, Aabid; Joshua Kangas; Luis Pedro Coelho; Shannon Quinn; Robert F Murphy (2010). "Automated image analysis for high-content screening and analysis". Journal of Biomolecular Screening. doi:10.1177/1087057110370894

Biomechanics

Biomechanics is concerned with the study of biological systems, at all levels of organization from cell organelles to the organism level. This chapter closely examines the crucial concepts of biomechanics, such as statics, dynamics, kinematics and kinetics as well as the domains of nanobiomechanics, plant and sports biomechanics, among others.

Biomechanics is the field of study that makes use of the laws of physics and engineering concepts to describe motion of body segments, and the internal and external forces, which act upon them during activity.

One objective of biomechanics is to determine the internal forces in muscles, tendons, bones and joints that arise within the human body due to interaction of external forces, gravitational forces on the body segments, and body posture. These internal forces are then used to explain the relationship between external environments and the internal injuries and tissue stresses.

Sports biomechanics explores the relationship between the body motion, internal forces and external forces to optimize the sport performance.

Biomechanics often applies modeling approach to understand the internal reaction forces in a body part of interest. Models of body segments are developed at varying degree of details depending upon the objective of the study. Modeling requires data about the size, mass and inertial properties of human body segments, and tissue strength limits (of muscles, bones, cartilages, tendons, ligaments etc.). Scientists have extensively studied such data on human internal structure and strength employing experimental study, cadaver dissection, X-rays, CT scans, and MRI.

Depending upon the detailing level of biomechanical modeling, it can employ complex mathematical and engineering principles. However, simple biomechanical models of human structure can help us to understand how the internal stresses are developed, and its interaction with the external environment. Biomechanics uses the principles of mechanics.

Newton's Laws of Mechanics

1. A body will maintain its stationary (or moving) state, until and unless, a net force is applied to it that changes its state.

2. When a net force 'F' is applied to a body of mass 'm', it changes the body's acceleration by 'a'. These three quantities are related to each other by the equation $F = m * a$.

3. Each force has an equal and opposite reaction force.

The standard international (SI) unit of force is one Newton, which is the amount of force required to change the acceleration by 1 meter/secon2 of a mass of 1 kg.

Force Vector

Force is a vector quantity, that is, it requires two quantities to describe it. One is the magnitude of the force and the other is the direction to which it is acting. Examples of other vector quantities are velocity and acceleration. As opposed to this, mass and distance are scalar quantities because they need only magnitude to describe them but no direction is necessary.

Graphically a force is represented by an arrow, the length of the arrow represents the magnitude and the direction of the arrow provides the direction of the force.

Resultant of Multiple Forces

Since the force have magnitude and direction, the magnitude of the forces acting on a point in the same direction only can be added numerically to obtain the magnitude of the resultant force. But if the forces have different directions, they cannot be added numerically to obtain the magnitude of the resultant force. Figure below shows the concept in a two dimensional situation. If the two forces 2N and 4N acts on the square block on one point and are parallel to each other then, the equivalent amount of force, which is called resultant force acting on the block at the same point, is 6N. But if the forces 2N and 4N are acting on different directions, then their resultant will not be 6N.

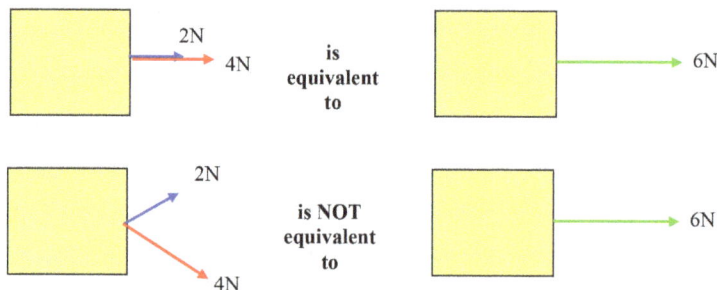

Figure: Forces are vector quantity. Their magnitudes cannot be numerically summed up to get the magnitude of the resultant force, unless they are concurrent and parallel.

Force Parallelogram

When two forces are not parallel to each other, we can draw a force parallelogram to obtain the magnitude and direction of the resultant force. Two parallel lines to the force vectors F1=4N and F2=2N are drawn graphically to form a parallelogram. The diagonal line of the parallelogram from the point of action of the two forces represents the resultant force vector. If the force vector lines are drawn to the scale then the magnitude and direction of the resultant force vector can now be measured directly from the graphics.

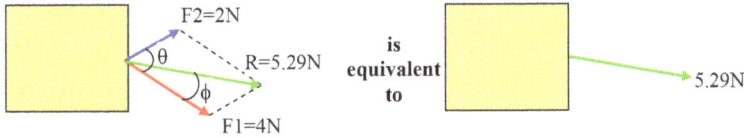

Figure: Force parallelogram method of finding resultant of two concurrent forces.

If there are three force vectors acting on a point (concurrent), then by taking any two forces we can first find the resultant of the two. Now using the resultant force vector of the two and the third force vector, we can draw a new parallelogram. The diagonal of this parallelogram would then represent the resultant of the three forces.

The magnitude and direction of two concurrent forces can also be determined from the formula given below. This formula can be derived using basic geometry. In the formula, θ is the angle between the two forces and ϕ being the angle between the resultant force and the F1 force. Let us apply the formula to find the resultant for our previous example forces of 4N and 2N. Let us also assume that the angle between the two forces $\theta = 60°$.

$$R = \sqrt{F_1^2 + F_2^2 + 2F_1F_2 \cos(\theta)} = \sqrt{2^2 + 4^2 + 2*2*4*\cos(60)} = \sqrt{4+16+16*1/2} = \sqrt{28} = 5.29 \ N$$

$$\phi = \tan^{-1}\left(\frac{F_2 \sin(\theta)}{F_1 + F_2 \cos(\theta)}\right) = \tan^{-1}\left(\frac{2\sin(60)}{4 + 2\cos(60)}\right) = \tan^{-1}\left(\frac{2*\sqrt{3/2}}{4+2*1/2}\right) = \tan^{-1}(0.346) = 19.1°$$

The magnitude of resultant R came out to be 5.29 N and the angle ϕ of the resultant from the F1 force (F1 = 4N in this case) came out to be 19.1°.

The above method of graphically drawing force parallelogram can be time consuming and complicated. Also the formula method allows us only to add two forces at a time.

Resolving Forces into Two Orthogonal Components

Any force vector F can be resolved into two orthogonal (perpendicular) components. Usually the two orthogonal directions are denoted as X and Y, and X being the horizontal and Y being the vertical direction. These two directions X and Y are also called X axis and Y axis. The simple formulae for the resolution are $F_x = F \cos(\theta)$ and $F_x = F \sin(\theta)$. Here, θ is the angle of the force vector F from positive X axis. We have to follow a sign convention for specifying this angle. When the angle from the positive X axis to the force is counterclockwise (CCW), the angle is positive. If it is clockwise (CW) the angle is negative.

The force F1 = 4N makes an angle 30° CW from the positive Xaxis. This means the angle $\theta 1 = -30°$. Applying the above formula, the X and Y components of this force are:

$$F1_x = 4\cos(-30°) = 4(0.866) = 3.46 \text{ N}$$
$$F1_y = 4\sin(-30°) = 4(-0.5) = -2 \text{ N}$$

$F1_y$ comes out to be negative. That means this force is directed towards the negative Y axis, which is vertically downward.

Similarly, the force F2 = 2N is also resolved into X and Y components. F2 is making an angle 30° with positive X axis, thus the angle $\theta 2 = 30°$, and

$$F2_x = 2\cos(30°) = 2(0.866) = 1.73 \text{ N}$$
$$F2_y = 2\sin(30°) = 2(0.5) = 1 \text{ N}$$

Figure below shows the forces 4N and 2N and their X and Y components. Notice that the X and Y components of a force make two sides of a rectangle, whose diagonal is the force that is being resolved. Rectangle is also a parallelogram. This means that the vector sum of the X and Y components of a force will produce the resultant equal to the force. That means a force is equivalent to the vector sum of its X and Y components, and vice versa.

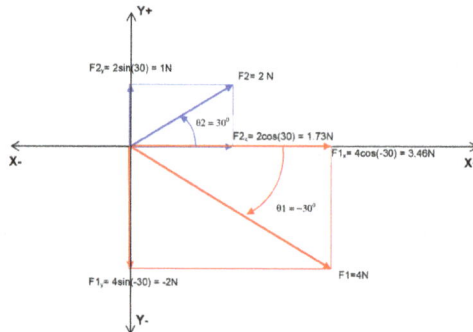

Figure: Resolving forces into its X and Y components

Finding Resultant of a System of Forces from their X and Y Components

If there is a system of concurrent forces, we can resolve each one into its X and Y components. Now as all X components are now in the same direction, we can numerically add their magnitudes together to obtain the resultant X component. We can treat all Y components in the same way.

$$F_x = F1_x + F2_x + F3_x + F4_x + F5_x + F6_x + \ldots$$
$$F_y = F1_y + F2_y + F3_y + F4_y + F5_y + F6_y + \ldots$$

Finally we can find the resultant F, of all forces, by finding the resultant of the Fx, and Fy force. Because Fx and Fy forces are at 90 to each other, the formulae for the magnitude F of the resultant and direction ϕ becomes (angle of the resultant from X axis) much simpler.

$$F = \sqrt{F_X^2 + F_Y^2} \quad \text{and} \quad \phi = \tan^{-1} \frac{F_Y}{F_X}$$

For our example problem,

$$Fx = F1_x + F2_x = 4\cos(-30°) + 2\cos(30°) = 4(0.866) + 2(0.866) = 3.46 + 1.73 = 5.19 \text{ N}$$
$$Fy = F1_y + F2_y = 4\sin(-30°) + 2\sin(30°) = 4(-0.5) + 2(0.5) = -2 + 1 = -1 \text{ N}$$

Then,

$$F = \sqrt{F_X^2 + F_Y^2} = \sqrt{5.19^2 + (-1)^2} = \sqrt{26.9316 + 1} = \sqrt{27.9361} = 5.29 \text{ N}$$
$$and \quad \phi = \tan^{-1} \frac{F_Y}{F_X} = \tan^{-1} \frac{(-1)}{5.19} = \tan^{-1}(-0.1927) = 10.91°$$

Graphically the above operations are shown in the figure given below. The figure also shows that if we find the resultant by the parallelogram method or by resolution method we get the same resultant force $F = 5.29 \text{ N}$.

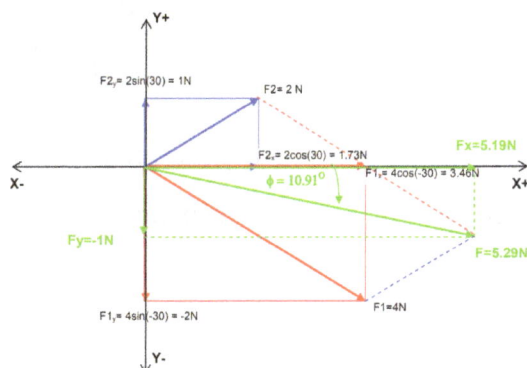

Figure: Vector sum of two forces from the resolved forces in X and Y directions.

Moment of a Force about a Point

If a force F acts on a body at a point A as shown in figure, then it produces a moment, $M = \bar{d} * F$ around another point B, which is at a (perpendicular) distance $\bar{d}$ from the line of action of the force. If we pin the body at point B, this moment M will try to rotate the body around pin. If the line of action of the force passes through the point B, then $\bar{d} = 0$ and the moment becomes zero. Thus moment of a force about a point on the line of action of the force is always zero.

Moment is also a vector quantity. In two dimensions, it is either CCW or CW. If one is treated as positive the other becomes negative.

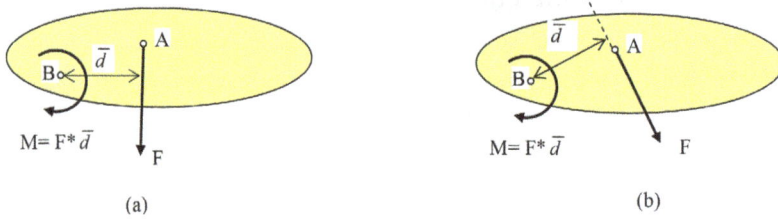

(a)   (b)

Figure: Moment of a force

For calculating moment of an inclined force, it is customary to resolve the force into X and Y components and then to find the moments due to Fx and Fy. If we know the horizontal and vertical distances between the points A and B, say x and y respectively then the moment at point B becomes:

$$M = M_x + M_y = -y*F_x + x*F_y$$

Suppose a force F = 10 N passes through the point A, whose horizontal (x) and vertical (y) distances from point B is 5 and 2 meters, respectively. F is inclined 60° CW with positive X axis. According to our sign convention of angles it is a negative angle. Then the magnitude of Fx and Fy are

$$F_x = 10\cos(-60°) = 10(0.5) = 5\,N$$

$$F_y = 10\sin(-60°) = 10(-0.866) = -8.66\,N$$

$$M = M_x + M_y = -y*F_x + x*F_y = (-2*5) + 5*(-8.66) = -10 - 43.3 = -53.3\,N-m.$$

Thus the moment of this inclined force at point B is 33.3 N-m in CW direction.

The above method of calculation of moment is explained graphically in the figure given below.

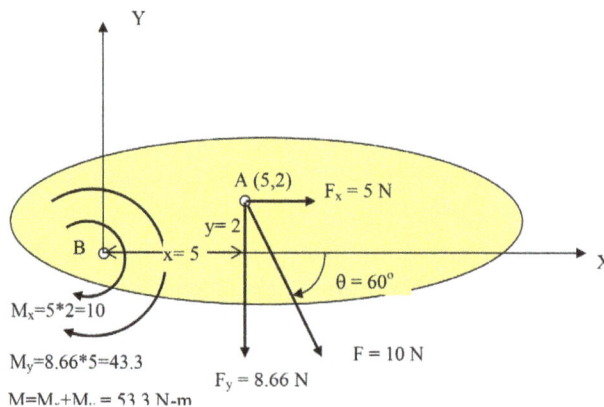

Figure: Calculation of the moment of an inclined force from its X and Y components.

Condition of Static Equilibrium and Free Body Diagram

If a net force acts on a static body, then according to Newton's laws of motion, the body must start moving. If the body doesn't move, it means that some internal forces and moments have developed, that are opposing the external forces and are keeping the body static. These internal forces and moments that are developed due to the external forces and moments, and that resist any motion of a static body, are called reaction forces and reaction moments, respectively.

Essentially, to maintain static equilibrium of a body both the following conditions must be satisfied.

(i) The sum total of all forces (both external and internal) acting on a body in any given direction must be equal to zero. In a 2D situation, this gives us two conditions that must be met.

$$(a)\ \sum F_x = 0 \quad \text{and} \quad (b)\ \sum F_y = 0$$

(ii) The sum total all moments (both due to external and internal forces) about any point on the body must be equal to zero. That is $\sum M = 0$.

For static conditions, most of the times, we can draw a free body diagram of the object we want to analyze. Free body diagram contains all known external forces and unknown internal forces. Then we use the equilibrium conditions, and solve for the unknown internal (reaction) forces and moments.

Example 1. A beam of 20 N weight is attached to a wall by means of a hinge and is supported by a cable from the roof. At the free end, it supports a vertically downward force of 300 N. The pertinent dimensions of the beam are shown in Figure below. If the beam is rigid, what forces will be developed at the hinge and the cable.

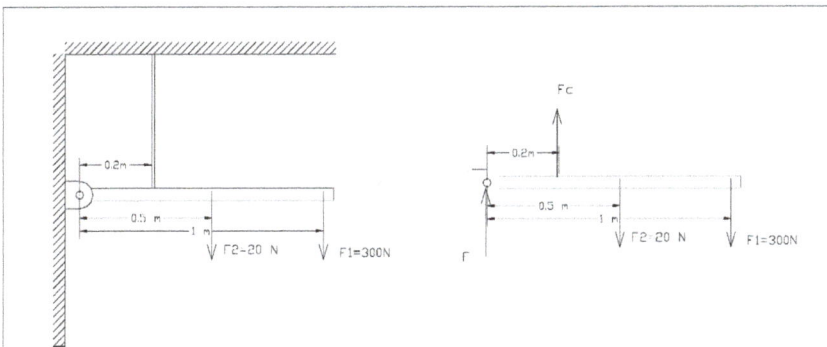

Solution: We can guess that the hinge and cable is giving upward forces on the beam, which are the internal forces with unknown values. We draw a free body diagram of the beam, with both known and unknown forces then apply the equilibrium conditions.

- $\sum F_x = 0$: It does not yield anything as there is no force in X direction.

- $\sum F_y = 0$: $Fc + F - 20 - 300 = 0$, i.e. $Fc + F = 320$

- $\sum M = 0$:   *Taking a moment at the left hinge point*

  $Fc(.2) - 20(.5) - 300(1) = 0, i.e..2Fc = 310 i.e., Fc = 310/.2 = 1550 N$

Then from equation $\sum F_y = 0$ $Fc + F - 20 - 300 = 0$, i.e. $Fc + F = 320$,

  F = 320 -1550 = -1230 N

We see that the force F at the hinge joint is -1230N. This means the direction of the force is in the negative Y direction that is downward. The cable will apply an upward force of 1150 N.

Body System Static Models

Using similar approach as described above we can estimate internal reaction forces developed at the body joints, and internal forces developed by the muscles to maintain the static equilibrium.

A two dimensional back model

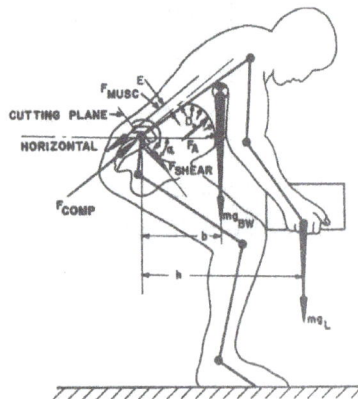

Figure: Simple cantilever low-back model of lifting

Load in hand mgL= 450 N

Upper body weight mg BW = 350 N

E = lever arm of erector spinae muscle =6.5 cm

h = distance of the load from L5/S1= 30 cm

b = distance of the upper body center of gravity from L5/S1 joint =20 cm

α = Upper body angle with horizontal = 55°

Find, the muscle force F_M , Spine compressive force Fc, and spine shear force Fs.

Solution:

Taking a moment around L5/S1 joint and equating it to Zero, we get

$$\sum M = 0 : FM * 6.5 - 350 * 20 - 450 * 30 = 0$$

Or, $F_M = (350 * 20 + 450 * 30)/6.5 = 3154$ N (downward)

That is the muscle has to produce a 3154 N force to maintain static equilibrium.

Resolving the body weight and force in hand into X and Y components,

$$F_{BWx} = F_{BW} \cos(\alpha) = 350 \cos(-55) = 201 \text{ N} \text{ (towards positive X direction)}$$
$$F_{BWy} = F_{BW} \sin(\alpha) = 350 \sin(-55) = -287 \text{ N} \text{ (towards negative Y direction)}$$

$$F_{Lx} = F_L \cos(\alpha) = 450 \cos(-55) = 258 \text{ N} \text{ (towards positive X direction)}$$
$$F_{Ly} = F_L \sin(\alpha) = 450 \sin(-55) = -369 \text{ N} \text{ (towards negative Y direction)}$$

Then, equating forces in Y directions,

$$\sum F_y = 0: \qquad \text{Fc} = 3154 + 287 + 369 = 3810 \text{ N}$$

Similarly, equating forces in X directions,

$$\sum F_x = \qquad F_s = 201 + 258 = 459 \text{ N}$$

Dynamics

Dynamics is the branch of physical science and subdivision of mechanics that is concerned with the motion of material objects in relation to the physical factors that affect them: force, mass, momentum, energy.

Dynamics can be subdivided into kinematics, which describes motion, without regard to its causes, in terms of position, velocity, and acceleration; and kinetics, which is concerned with the effect of forces and torques on the motion of bodies having mass. The foundations of dynamics were laid at the end of the 16th century by Galileo Galilei who, by experimenting with a smooth ball rolling down an inclined plane, derived the law of motion for falling bodies; he was also the first to recognize that force is the cause of changes in the velocity of a body, a fact formulated by Isaac Newton in the 17th century in his second law of motion. This law states that the force acting on a body is equal to the rate of change of the body's momentum.

Two Major Areas

- Bone Remodeling - This is a slow process (couple months) but is the reality whenever you introduce a static element, like an artificial hip, in conjunction with living bone. The stiffness of the artificial component impacts the force distribution in the bone, where the bone reallocates density to match that stiffness. This can result in failure of the bone, usually underneath the artificial component. Also, modeling of the artificial component to match the anti-fatigue properties of living bone, usually on the order of years. Modeling bone as static, in applications with implants - historically, this is a disaster since the first artificial knee (sliding joint, not hinge) during the Civil War.

- Non-linear movement - For artificial limbs when positioning with mass. Moving a hand to grab a cup of liquid and bring to mouth, for example. If you do this with linear motion, it takes forever! - compared with a natural arm completing the same trajectory. This type of control system was first introduced for the space shuttle arm but clearly is the same kind of dynamic control problem - at the expected reduction in scale. Same thing with ambulatory control. Walking after picking up a back back, shifting balance to meet an incline, etc. Being able to do this in real-time, at natural velocities - all dynamics, with appropriate control systems. Shifting from walking to running - long way to go here as well.

Statics

Statics is the study of the forces acting on a body at rest or moving with a constant velocity. Although the human body is almost always accelerating, a static analysis offers a simple method of addressing musculoskeletal problems. This analysis may either solve the problem or provide a basis for a more sophisticated dynamic analysis.

Newton's Laws

Since the musculoskeletal system is simply a series of objects in contact with each other, some of the basic physics principles developed by Sir Isaac Newton are useful. Newton's laws are as follows:

First law: An object remains at rest (or continues moving at a constant velocity) unless acted upon by an unbalanced external force.

Second law: If there is an unbalanced force acting on an object, it produces an acceleration in the direction of the force, directly proportional to the force $(f = ma)$.

Third law: For every action (force) there is a reaction (opposing force) of equal magnitude but in the opposite direction.

From the first law, it is clear that if a body is at rest, there can be no unbalanced external forces acting on it. In this situation, termed static equilibrium, all of the external forces acting on a body must add (in a vector sense) to zero. An extension of this law to objects larger than a particle is that the sum of the external moments acting on that body must also be equal to zero for the body to be at rest. Therefore, for a three-dimensional analysis, there are a total of six equations that must be satisfied for static equilibrium:

$$\sum F_X = 0 \quad \sum F_Y = 0 \quad \sum F_Z = 0$$
$$\sum M_X = 0 \quad \sum M_Y = 0 \quad \sum M_Z = 0$$

For a two-dimensional analysis, there are only two in-plane force components and one perpendicular moment (torque) component:

$$\sum F_X = 0 \quad \sum F_Y = 0 \quad \sum M_Z = 0$$

Under many conditions, it is reasonable to assume that all body parts are in a state of static equilibrium and these three equations can be used to calculate some of the forces acting on the musculoskeletal system. When a body is not in static equilibrium, Newton's second law states that any unbalanced forces and moments are proportional to the acceleration of the body.

Solving Problems

A general approach used to solve for forces during static equilibrium is as follows:

Step 1   Isolate the body of interest.

Step 2   Sketch this body and all external forces (referred to as a free body diagram).

Step 3   Sum the forces and moments equal to zero.

Step 4   Solve for the unknown forces.

As a simple example, consider the two 1-kg balls hanging from strings shown in Box. What is the force acting on the top string? Although this is a very simple problem that can be solved by inspection, a formal analysis is presented. Step 1 is to sketch the entire system and then place a dotted box around the body of interest. Consider a box that encompasses both balls and part of the string above the top one.

Proceeding to step 2, a free body diagram is sketched. As indicated by Newton's first law, only external forces are considered for these analyses. For this example, everything inside the dotted box is considered part of the body of interest. External forces are caused by the contact of two objects, one inside the box and one outside the box. In this example, there are three external forces: tension in the top string and the weight of each of the balls.

Why is the tension on the top string considered an external force, but not the force on the bottom string? The reason is that the tension on the top string is an external force (part of the string is in the box and part is outside the box), and the force on the bottom string is an internal force (the entire string is located inside the box). This is a very important distinction because it allows for isolation of the forces on specific muscles or joints in the musculoskeletal system.

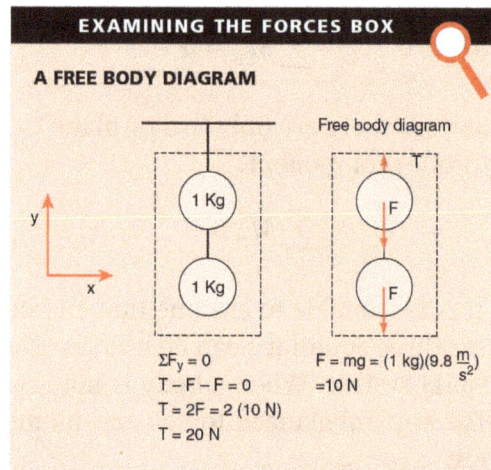

EXAMINING THE FORCES BOX

A FREE BODY DIAGRAM

Free body diagram

$\Sigma F_y = 0$

$T - F - F = 0$

$T = 2F = 2\ (10\ N)$

$T = 20\ N$

$F = mg = (1\ kg)(9.8\ \frac{m}{s^2})$

$= 10\ N$

Why the weight of each ball is considered an external force? Although gravity is not caused by contact between two objects, it is caused by the interaction of two objects and is treated in the same manner as a contact force. One of the objects is inside the box (the ball) and the other is outside the box (the Earth). In general, as long as an object is located within the box, the force of gravity acting on it should be considered an external force.

Why the weight of the string is not considered an external force? To find an exact answer to the problem, it should be considered. However, since its weight is far less than that of the balls, it is considered negligible. In biomechanical analyses, assumptions are often made to ignore certain forces, such as the weight of someone's watch during lifting.

Once all the forces are in place, step 3 is to sum all the forces and moments equal to zero. There are no forces in the x direction, and since all of the forces pass through the same point, there are no moments to consider. That leaves only one equation: sum of the forces in the y direction equal to zero. The fourth and final step is to solve for the unknown force. The mass of the balls is converted to force by multiplying by the acceleration of gravity. The complete analysis is shown in Box.

Simple Musculoskeletal Problems

Although most problems can be addressed with the above approach, there are special situations in which a problem is simplified. These may be useful both for solving problems analytically and for quick assessment of clinical problems from a biomechanical perspective.

Linear Forces

The simplest type of system, linear forces, consists of forces with the same orientation and line of action. The only things that can be varied are the force magnitudes and directions. An example is provided in Box. Notice that the only equation needed is summing the forces along the y axis equal to zero. When dealing with linear forces, it is best to align either the x or y axis with the orientation of the forces.

Parallel Forces

A slightly more complicated system is one in which all the forces have the same orientation but not the same line of action. In other words, the force vectors all run parallel to each other. In this situation, there are still only forces along one axis, but there are moments to consider as well.

Levers

A lever is an example of a parallel force system that is very common in the musculoskeletal system. Although not all levers contain parallel forces, that specific case is focused on here. A basic understanding of this concept allows for a rudimentary analysis of a biomechanical problem with very little mathematics.

A lever consists of a rigid body with two externally applied forces and a point of rotation. In general, for the musculoskeletal joint, one of the forces is produced by a muscle, one force is provided by contact with the environment (or by gravity) and the point of rotation is the center of rotation of the joint. The two forces can either be on the same side or different sides of the center of rotation (COR).

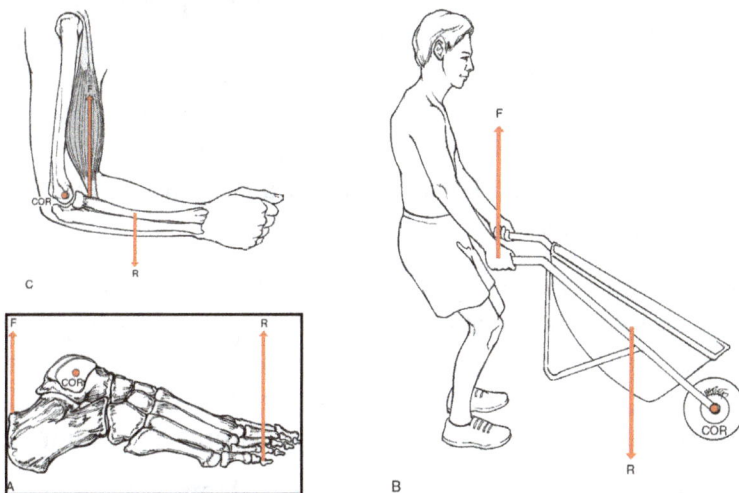

Figure: Classification of lever systems. Examples of the three different classes of levers, where F is the exerted force, R is the reaction force, and COR is the center of rotation. Most musculoskeletal joints behave as third class levers. A. First class lever. B. Second class lever. C. Third class lever.

If the forces are on different sides of the COR, the system is considered a first class lever. If the forces are on the same side of the COR and the external force is closer to the COR than the muscle force, it is a second class lever. If the forces are on the same side of the COR and the muscle force is closer to the COR than the external force, it is a third class lever. There are several cases of first class levers; however, most joints in the human body behave as third class levers. Second class levers are almost never observed within the body. Examples of all three levers are given in Figure 1.9.

If moments are summed about the COR for any lever, the resistive force is equal to the muscle force times the ratio of the muscle and resistive moment arms:

$$F_R = F_M \times (MA_M / MA_R)$$

The ratio of the muscle and resistive moment arms (MA_M / MA_R) is referred to as the mechanical advantage of the lever. Based on this equation and the definition of levers, the mechanical advantage is greater than one for a second class lever, less than one for a third class lever, and either for a first class lever. A consequence of this is that since most joints behave as third class levers, muscle forces must always be greater than the force of the resistive load they are opposing. Although this may appear to represent an inefficient design, muscles sacrifice their mechanical advantage to produce large motions and high-velocity motions. This equation is also valid in cases where the two forces are not parallel, as long as their moment arms are known.

Center of Gravity and Stability

Another example of a parallel force system is the use of the center of gravity to determine stability. The center of gravity of an object is the point at which all of the weight of that body can be thought to be concentrated, and it depends on a body's shape and mass distribution. The center of gravity of the human body in the anatomical position is approximately at the level of the second sacral vertebra . This location changes as the shape of the body is altered. When a person bends forward, his or her center of gravity shifts anteriorly and inferiorly. The location of the center of gravity is also affected by body mass distribution changes. For example, if a person were to develop more leg muscle mass, the center of mass would shift inferiorly.

The location of a person's center of gravity is important in athletics and other fast motions because it simplifies the use of Newton's second law. More important from a clinical point of view is the effect of the center of gravity on stability. For motions in which the acceleration is negligible, it can be shown with Newton's first law that the center of gravity must be contained within a person's base of support to maintain stability.

Consider the situation of a person concerned about falling forward. Assume for the moment that there is a ground reaction force at his toes and heel. When he is standing upright, his center of gravity is posterior to his toes, so there is a counterclockwise moment at his toes. This is a stable position, since the moment can be balanced by the ground reaction force at his heel. If he bends forward at his hips to touch the ground and leans too far forward, his center of gravity moves anterior to his toes and the weight of his upper body produces a clockwise moment at his toes. Since there is no further anterior support, this moment is unbalanced and the man will fall forward. However, if in addition to hip flexion he plantarflexes at his ankles while keeping his knee straight, he is in a stable position with his center of gravity posterior to his toes.

Advanced Musculoskeletal Problems

One of the most common uses of static equilibrium applied to the musculoskeletal system is to solve for unknown muscle forces. This is a very useful tool because as mentioned above, there are currently no noninvasive experimental methods that can be used to measure in vivo muscle forces. There are typically 3 types of forces to consider in a musculoskeletal problem: (a) the joint reaction force between the two articular surfaces, (b) muscle forces and (c) forces due to the body's interaction with the outside world. So how many unknown parameters are associated with these forces? To answer this, the location of all of the forces with their points of application must be identified. For the joint reaction force nothing else is known, so there are two unknown parameters: magnitude and orientation. The orientation of a muscle force can be measured, so there is one unknown parameter, magnitude. Finally, any force interaction with the outside world can theoretically be measured, possibly with a handheld dynamometer or by knowing the weight of the segment, so there are no unknown parameters.

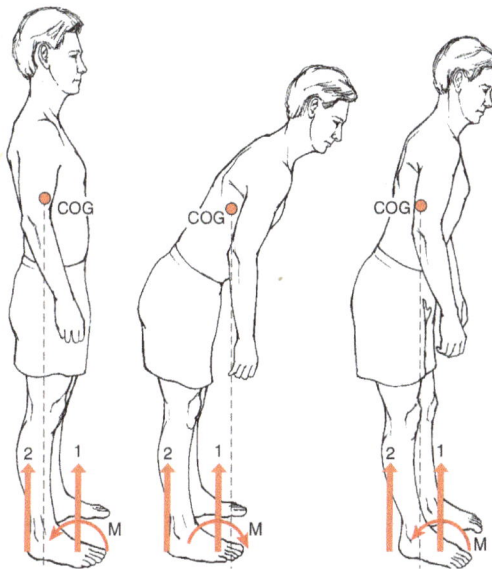

Figure: Center of gravity.

For the man in the figure to maintain his balance, his center of gravity must be maintained within his base of support. This is not a problem in normal standing (A). When he bends over at the waist, however, his center of gravity may shift anterior to the base of support, creating an unstable situation (B). The man needs to plantarflex at the ankles to maintain his balance (C).

Consequently, there are two unknown parameters for the joint reaction force and one unknown parameter for each muscle. However, there are only three equations available from a two-dimensional analysis of Newton's first law. Therefore, if there is more than one muscle force to consider, there are more unknown parameters than available equations. This situation is referred to as statically indeterminate, and there are an infinite number of possible solutions. To avoid this problem, only one muscle force can be considered. Although this is an oversimplification of most musculoskeletal situations, solutions based on a single muscle can provide a general perspective of the requirements of a task.

TABLE: Body Segment Parameters Derived from Dempster

	Percentage of Total Body Weight (%)	Location of the Center of Mass (% of limb segment length from proximal end)	Moment of Inertia about the Center of Mass (kg X m^2)
Head and neck	7.9	43.3	0.029
Trunk	48.6	n.a.	n.a.
Upper extremity	4.9	51.2^a	0.335
Arm	2.7	43.6	0.040
Forearm and hand	2.2	67.7	0.058
Forearm	1.6	43.0	0.018
Hand	0.6	50.6^b	0.002
Lower extremity	15.7	43.4^c	1.785
Thigh	9.6	43.3	0.298
Leg and foot	5.9	43.3	0.339
Leg	4.5	43.4	0.143
Foot	1.4	43.8^d	0.007

a Measured from axis of shoulder to ulnar styloid process.
b Measured to PIP joint of long finger.
c Measured to medial malleolus.
d Measured from heel.

Force Analysis with a Single Muscle

There are additional assumptions that are typically made to solve for a single muscle force:

- Two-dimensional analysis

- No deformation of any tissues

- No friction in the system

- The single muscle force that has been selected can be concentrated in a single line of action

- No acceleration

The glenohumeral joint is used as an example to help demonstrate the general strategy for approaching these problems. Since only one muscle force can be considered, the supraspinatus is chosen for analysis. The same general approach introduced earlier in this chapter for addressing a system in static equilibrium is used.

Step one is to isolate the body of interest, which for this problem is the humerus. In step two, a free body diagram is drawn, with all of the external forces clearly labeled: the weight of the arm (F_G), the supraspinatus force (F_S), and the glenohumeral joint reaction force (F_J). Note that external objects like the scapula are often included in the free body diagram to make the diagram complete. However, the scapula is external to the analysis and is only included for convenience. It is important to keep track of which objects are internal and which ones are external to the isolated body.

The next step is to sum the forces and moments to zero to solve for the unknown values. Since the joint reaction force acts through the COR, a good strategy is to start by summing the moments to zero at that point. This effectively eliminates the joint reaction force from this equation because its moment arm is equal to zero. The forces along the x and y axes are summed to zero to find those components of the joint reaction force. The fourth and final step is to solve for the unknown parameters in these three equations. In this example, the magnitude of the supraspinatus force is 203 N, and the joint reaction force is 203 N laterals and 28 N superior. Those components represent the force of the scapula acting on the humerus. Newton's third law can then be used to find the force of the humerus acting on the scapula: 203 N medial and 28 N inferior.

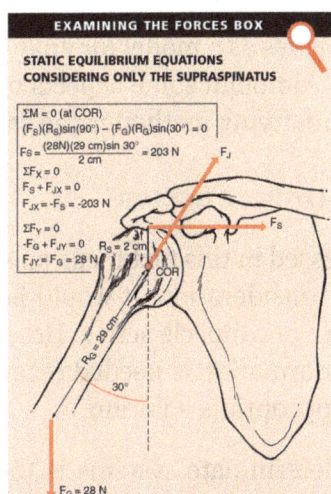

EXAMINING THE FORCES BOX

STATIC EQUILIBRIUM EQUATIONS
CONSIDERING ONLY THE SUPRASPINATUS

$\Sigma M = 0$ (at COR)

$(F_S)(R_S)\sin(90°) - (F_G)(R_G)\sin(30°) = 0$

$F_S = \dfrac{(28N)(29\ cm)\sin 30°}{2\ cm} \approx 203\ N$

$\Sigma F_X = 0$

$F_S + F_{JX} = 0$

$F_{JX} = -F_S = -203\ N$

$\Sigma F_Y = 0$

$-F_G + F_{JY} = 0 \quad R_S = 2\ cm$

$F_{JY} = F_G = 28\ N$

$R_G = 29\ cm$

$30°$

$F_G = 28\ N$

Note that the muscle force is much larger than the weight of the arm. This is expected, considering the small moment arm of the muscle compared with the moment arm of the force due to gravity. While this puts muscles at a mechanical disadvantage for force production, it enables them to amplify their motion. For example, a 1-cm contraction of the supraspinatus results in a 20-cm motion at the hand.

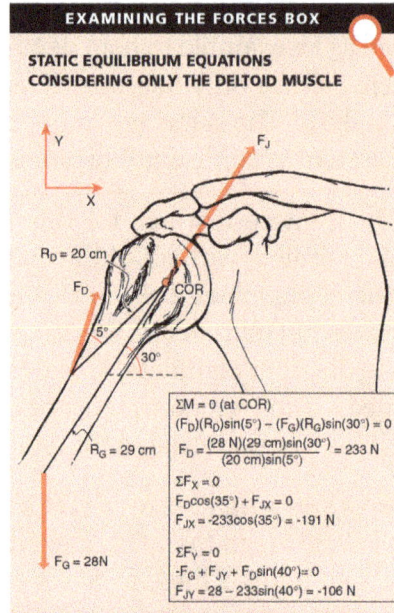

EXAMINING THE FORCES BOX

STATIC EQUILIBRIUM EQUATIONS CONSIDERING ONLY THE DELTOID MUSCLE

$\Sigma M = 0$ (at COR)

$(F_D)(R_D)\sin(5°) - (F_G)(R_G)\sin(30°) = 0$

$F_D = \dfrac{(28 \text{ N})(29 \text{ cm})\sin(30°)}{(20 \text{ cm})\sin(5°)} = 233 \text{ N}$

$\Sigma F_X = 0$

$F_D\cos(35°) + F_{JX} = 0$

$F_{JX} = -233\cos(35°) = -191 \text{ N}$

$\Sigma F_Y = 0$

$-F_G + F_{JY} + F_D\sin(40°) = 0$

$F_{JY} = 28 - 233\sin(40°) = -106 \text{ N}$

The problem can be solved again by considering the middle deltoid instead of the supraspinatus. For those conditions, the above box shows that the deltoid muscle force is 233 N and the force of the humerus acting on the scapula is 191 N medial and 106 N superior. Notice that although the force required of each muscle is similar (supraspinatus, 203 N vs. deltoid, 230 N), the deltoid generates a much higher superior force and the supraspinatus generates a much higher medial force.

The analysis presented above serves as a model for analyzing muscle and joint reaction forces in subsequent chapters. Although some aspects of the problem will clearly vary from joint to joint, the basic underlying method is the same.

Force Analysis with Multiple Muscles

Although most problems addressed in this text focus on solving for muscle forces when only one muscle is taken into consideration, it would be advantageous to solve problems in which there is more than one muscle active. However such systems are statically indeterminate. Additional information is needed regarding the relative contribution of each muscle to develop an appropriate solution.

One method for analyzing indeterminate systems is the optimization method. Since an indeterminate system allows an infinite number of solutions, the optimization approach helps select the "best" solution. An optimization model minimizes some cost function to produce a single solution. This function may be the total force in all of the muscles or possibly the total stress (force/area) in all of the muscles. While it might make sense that the central nervous system attempts to minimize the work it has to do to perform a function, competing demands of a joint must also be met. For example, in the glenohumeral example above, it might be most efficient from a force production standpoint to assume that the deltoid acts alone. However, from a stability standpoint, the contribution of the rotator cuff is essential.

Another method for analyzing indeterminate systems is the reductionist model in which a set of rules is applied for the relative distribution of muscle forces based on electro-myographic (EMG) signals. One approach involves developing these rules on the basis of the investigator's subjective knowledge of EMG activity, anatomy, and physiological constraints . Another approach is to have subjects perform isometric contractions at different force levels while measuring EMG signals and to develop an empirical rela-tionship between EMG and force level. Perhaps the most common approach is based on the assumption that muscle force is proportional to its cross-sectional area and EMG level. This method has been attempted for many joints, such as the shoulder, knee and hip. One of the key assumptions in all these approaches is that there is a known rela-tionship between EMG levels and force production.

Kinematics

Movement and position are called kinematic variables. Kinematics also falls into two very clear categories: linear and angular. Linear kinematics is usually those associated with overall movement of an athlete (like running velocity or jumping height) and an-gular kinematics is those associated with the movement of specific joints.

Linear Kinematics

- Displacement – displacement is a change in position of an object. Jumping height is an example of a displacement that is often measured in biomechanics.

- Ground contact time – ground contact times are the durations of time in which feet are in contact with the ground during athletic movements, such as drop jumps or sprint running. Sprint running displays some of the shortest ground contact times, which are around 0.1 seconds, which does not allow much time for the athletes to exert force to propel themselves forwards.

- Flight time – flight times are the durations of time in which an athlete is not in contact with the ground during athletic movements, such as during vertical jumps or sprint running. During vertical jumps, flight time can be used to esti-mate jump height by using Newton's laws of motion.

- Velocity – velocity is the rate of change of position of an athlete (in m/s), which is the displacement divided by time. It is a vector quantity (meaning that it has a direction associated with it) and speed is its scalar equivalent.

- Acceleration – acceleration is the rate of change of velocity of an athlete (in m/s/s), which is the change in velocity divided by time. It is also vector quantity (meaning that it has a direction associated with it) and is proportional to both the external force exerted upon it and its mass.

Angular Kinematics

- Concentric – concentric muscle actions occur when muscles shorten under tension, leading to changes in joint position.

- Eccentric – eccentric muscle actions occur when muscles lengthen under tension, leading to changes in joint position.

- Isometric – isometric muscle actions occur when no movement in the joint take place. The muscle does shorten and the tendon does lengthen but this does not alter joint position.

- Range of motion (ROM) – the displacement in angular movement is generally measured by reference to ROM, which can be reported in either degrees or radians (rad).

- Center of mass (COM) – the center of mass is the unique point within an object where the weighted relative position of the distributed mass of the object sums to zero. In biomechanics, it is common to assume that an object behaves as if it were a point mass located at the COM rather than a distributed mass, for ease of calculations.

- Joint angular velocity – joint angular velocity is the rate of change of joint ROM, which is therefore measured in degrees/s or rad/s.

Kinetics

Force and moments are kinetic variables. Force in biomechanics is usually exerted either by muscles acting on joints or by heavy external objects (like barbells or the ground) acting on the human body. Kinetics falls into two very clear categories: linear and angular. Linear kinetics are usually those associated with overall forces exerted upon an athlete (like ground reaction forces during jumping) and angular kinetics are those associated with the turning forces at specific joints.

Linear Kinetics

- Force – force equals mass times acceleration ($F = ma$) and where mass (kg) and acceleration (m/s/s) are expressed in standard international (SI) units, force is automatically expressed in Newtons (N).

- Ground reaction force – When you jump, sprint, or perform an Olympic lift, you exert force into the ground. Force-plates measure these forces. During vertical jumping, most of the force produced is vertical. However, in sprinting, you have vertical forces as well as horizontal forces. When the foot strikes the ground during maximum speed sprinting, at first the force is projected forward which is called braking forces, and once the COM passes over the foot, the force is projected rearward which is called propulsive forces.

- Muscle force – when muscles contract or are stretched, they create muscle force. This muscle force pulls on bones which creates joint torque. In general, force, including muscle force, is measured in Newtons.

- Rate of force development (RFD) – RFD is the rate of change of force over time, expressed as N/s.

- Impulse – impulse is force multiplied by time over which the force acts, expressed as Ns.

- Work – work is force muiltiplied by the distance moved as a result of the force acting, expressed in Joules (J).

- Power – power is the rate at which work is done, and can be calculated either by dividing the work done by the time in which the work was done or by multiplying the force applied by the velocity at which it was applied1, expressed in Watts (W).

- Momentum – momentum is mass multiplied by velocity, expressed in kg m/s.

- Variable resistance – variable external resistance is a form of external resistance that changes throughout the movement. This can be achieved in practice using bands and chains in combination with barbells or by using machine weights with cam devices.

- Isokinetic resistance – isokinetic external resistance is a form of variable resistance that maintains the velocity of the movement constant irrespective of the force applied. It is only achievable in practice using a dynamometer.

- Accommodating resistance – strictly, accommodating resistance is the same as isokinetic resistance, where the load "accommodates" the force applied by the subject so that velocity remains constant throughout the movement. In practice, the term "accommodating resistance" is often used to refer to bands and chains, which are a form of variable resistance that approximate isokinetic external resistance.

- Isoinertial resistance – isoinertial external resistance is any external resistance that remains constant throughout the movement. Most typical free weight exercises are isoinertial, as the mass or loads do not change during the exercise.

Angular Kinetics

- Joint moment – a moment is the turning effect produced by a force. It is often synonymous with torque, which can be thought of as the rotational analog to linear force (turning force), and is calculated by multiplying the perpendicular force by the distance from the pivot (or axis of rotation).

- External joint moments – Resistance in strength training produces an external moment, whereas

- Internal joint moments – muscles produce an internal moment to counteract the external moment. Moments are usually measured in Newton-meters.

- Joint power – it is possible to measure the power output of individual joints during movement by multiplying the torque by the joint angular velocity. It is usually reported in Newton-meters per second.

- Rate of torque development (RTD) – and is usually measured in Newton-meters per second.

Plant Biomechanics

Mechanics is an inseparable feature of the abiotic interactions of plants with gravity, wind, soil, aquatic currents, and waves, and the biotic interactions with other plants, animals, and microorganisms through contact, impact, adhesion, penetration, catching, or propagule transport. Internally, mechanics is central to water transport, the 'power of growth', and cell–cell interactions.

Plant biomechanics can be defined simply as the study of the structures and functions of biological systems from the phylum *Plantae* by making use of concepts and methods from mechanics.

- Fluid mechanics: the branch of physics that studies how fluids flow under the influence of forces. It can be divided into fluid statics and fluid dynamics. Fluid mechanics is not only used in plant biomechanics to understand the interaction of plants with wind or other currents and the flow of internal saps, but also to understand the process of growth itself. The general framework used to model the behaviour of fluids comprises the Navier–Stokes equations.

- Fracture mechanics: the branch of mechanics that studies the propagation of cracks and bubbles in materials. Of specific concern is the influence of microscopic defects and crack 'growth' that lead to possible instabilities and subsequent catastrophic ruptures. Fracture mechanics has been applied to plant tissues and organs such as wood, leaf, and fruit tissues, in relation to wind-break function, or the effect of herbivory. It is also a central aspect in studying the biomechanics of invasive growth and root growth in soils.

- Growth: the term 'growth' is polysemic, and may lead to confusion when used in an interdisciplinary context. In plants, growth involves the deformation (strain) of existing polymeric cell walls, so measuring the intensity and spatial distribution of growth may require kinematical methods. Stressing of the cell wall to balance internal turgor pressure provides the power for growth. This internal pressure itself results from the reaction of the cell wall (as well as that of neighboring cells) to the entrance of water driven by osmotic differences in cell contents. However, at the same time, some new wall material is synthesized and added to the inner side of the existing cell wall or into a new cell wall if the cell undergoes cell division while expanding. Finally, the rheology of growing cell walls is usually anisotropic and can be regulated very rapidly in response to different cues, including mechanical ones. All these characteristics make the calculation of stress distribution in plant biomechanics very different from standard strength of material calculations as soon as growth needs to be taken into account.

- Hydraulics: a set of simplified models of fluid dynamics specifically adapted to a set of engineering situations such as pipe flow and river channels. Hydraulic models are relevant to many biological situations, e.g. sap conduction in xylem, but care should be taken when using them in plant systems.

- Instability: a situation where some output or internal state variable of a system varies greatly (through positive feedback) under small perturbations from the background mechanical noise. The system may thereby move from an unstable equilibrium state to another state of (stable) equilibrium or undergo rupture. For instance, in fracture mechanics, a crack can propagate without bounds when its length reaches a critical value. Similarly, in a fluid that is under tension (e.g. xylem sap), small gaseous bubbles can grow suddenly and boundlessly as soon as they reach a critical size, creating cavitation and embolism. On a different scale, in structural mechanics, a column under compression can become unstable when it exceeds a critical length. Any deflection of that column increases the lever arm on it, and hence the torque, which in turn increases deflection, and so on. This is called buckling or buckling instability. Both processes may be important to plant mechanical integrity and life. Instability is also a central aspect of fast active motion in plants, where the sudden release of accumulated elastic energy can be understood as an elastic instability.

- Integrative modeling: this is modeling that explicitly combines several mechanisms and usually deals with changes in scale. This integration relies on the theory of mechanics, and is at the heart of structural mechanics. Integrative modelling is thus a tool to interpret experiments, estimate non-observable variables such as stress, and identify the mechanisms driving a given phenomenon or trait. It has also been used to integrate the model of mechanosensing from the cell scale up to the organ scale.

- Kinematics: the quantitative and phenomenological study of the motion, deformation, and flow of bodies, without analyzing their causes. Kinematics is a central tool in studying the movement of plants and the quantitative analysis of growth and morphogenesis, allowing for a consistent spatiotemporal description of all the biophysical and biochemical processes involved, e.g. water and nutrient influxes, gene regulation, and protein synthesis.

- Mechanics of cellular solids: a developing branch of mechanics at the intersection between structural, continuum, and soft matter mechanics that focuses on the mechanical behavior of cellular materials. Many plant tissues have been described as cellular solids (e.g. parenchyma, sclerenchyma, wood), and quantitative links can be drawn between the microscopic anatomical layout of these tissues and their macroscopic mechanical function at the whole-tissue scale. For example, this approach has been used to analyze the strength of wood and the mechanical stability of plants in wind, the resistance of xylem conduits to collapse under the internal depression of the sap, and the behavior of meristems.

- Mechanism analysis: a mechanism is an assembly of bodies connected by joints that produces a force or motion transmission. Mechanism analysis has been used to study animal locomotion but is also relevant in some types of plant motion, such as fast motions.

- Nastic movement: active plant movement triggered by environmental stimuli (e.g. touch, temperature, humidity, or light irradiance) in which the direction of movement is not dependent on the direction of the stimulus. Some fast motions in plants are nastic movements, such as the closing of the Venus flytrap leaf when it captures prey or the folding of the mimosa leaf when it is disturbed. The mechanical energy for nastic motion can be provided by turgor pressure changes in elastic cells or through growth.

- Nutation: an active and autonomous helicoidal plant movement due to the successive bending of the organ in different directions while elongating. Whether or not this is related to gravitropism is a long-debated question. The amplitude of nutation is much larger in twining plants and is usually referred to as circumnutation.

- Rheology: the quantitative and qualitative study of the deformation and flow of matter (from the aphorism *ta panta rhei*: 'everything flows' from the philosophy of Heraclitus). Rheological studies lead to the definition of phenomenological models called 'constitutive laws' that relate stresses to strains and strain rates and potentially to other physical variables (e.g. temperature). The strength of the material, i.e. the limit of the constitutive equations, is also studied. Numerous studies of cell-wall, cell, and tissue rheology have been undertaken in plant biomechanics, in particular to understand the involvement of the cell wall in the control of expansion growth, morphogenesis, stiffness, and strength in plants.

- Soft matter and disordered media: states of matter that do not have the precise order of crystalline solids and are often intermediate between fluid and solid states. They include polymers, colloids, gels, vesicles, emulsions, foams, films, surfactants, micelles, suspensions, liquid crystals, and granular materials. Therefore, many biological materials fall in this category such as growing cell walls, cytoplasm, root and leaf exudates, cuticles, and soft tissues, as well as materials in the plant's environment like soil. In general, these states are characterized by mesoscopic structures (e.g. polymeric chains, chains of contacts between grains and force arches in granular solids, bubbles, or drops) that strongly influence their mechanical properties.

- Soft matter mechanics and rheology: mechanical and physical analysis of soft matter. Due to the existence of mesoscopic structures, soft matter displays mechanical properties that are intermediate between typical solids and fluids (such as non-linear rheology, flow thresholds, and internal relaxation time), which may lead to many instabilities, symmetry breaking, and pattern formation. Soft matter mechanics has reinvigorated fluid and solid mechanics and is being applied, for example, to plant growth and morphogenesis and to plant motion and tribology.

- Structural mechanics, Structural analysis: the branch of solid mechanics dealing with structures like beams, columns, plates, shells, and assemblies thereof (e.g. trees, trusses). In plants, principles of structural mechanics have been applied in order to mechanistically integrate the behaviour of: (i) macromolecules in a subcellular complex; (ii) cell walls in the behaviour of a tissue viewed as a cellular solid; (iii) tissues inside a complex organ; and (iv) a set of organs, such as the dynamics of a complex tree vibrating in the wind.

- Thigmomorphogenesis: the plant physiological response to external mechanical stimuli, which in natural conditions come mostly from the drag by wind or currents, raindrops, and the contact and rubbing by neighboring objects, plants, or passing animals (from the Greek word *thigma* meaning 'touch'). Thigmomorphogenesis was first demonstrated by submitting plants to artificial mechanical loads. A syndrome of responses is then observed in a large number of species, involving: (i) a reduction in longitudinal stem growth; (ii) a stimulation of secondary cambial growth (if present), possibly with differentiation of a more flexible but stronger 'flexure wood'; and (iii) a reallocation of biomass to the root system. This mechanosensitive control of growth allometries results in stunting and more anchored shoots, while conserving most of the capacity for wind drag reduction through reconfiguration made possible by the more flexible wood. The thigmomorphogenetic syndrome thus improves plant acclimation to its mechanical environment. Studies under natural conditions on isolated plants as well as on forest and crop dense stands have indeed shown that thigmomorphogenesis is a major process in the control of plant canopy growth in the ecological range of natural chronic winds or water currents.

- Toughness: Amount of mechanical energy (work) per volume that a material can absorb and/or dissipate before rupturing (unit $J/m3$). The toughness of a material depends on (i) the type and amount of defects existing in the material, and there possible control through mechanobiological wounding reactions, (ii) the balance between elastic and plastic deformation of the material depending on its content and ultrastructure, and (iii) the existence of crack-stopping anatomical features (holes and lumens, inclusions of soft materials). The study of the rheological and anatomical bases of toughness in plant is central to the understanding of the mechanical stability of plants and the resistance to pathogens or herbivory. It is also important for the use of plant-derived materials by animals and humans (e.g. texture and taste of fruits and vegetables, safety of wooden or bamboo constructions, and so on), and therefore studied in ecological and engineering sciences.

- Tribology: an interdisciplinary field at the intersection of mechanics, rheology, soft matter sciences, and chemistry that studies the phenomena of friction, adhesion, cohesion, abrasion, erosion, and corrosion at the interfaces between the surfaces of two systems. In plant biomechanics, tribology may be essential in understanding, for example, lubrication in root growth, cell-to-cell adhesion, insect-to-leaf adhesion, and insect trapping.

Plant systems that might by studied from a biomechanical perspective range from molecular and cellular structures (like DNA, stretch-activated channels, the cytoskeleton, cell membranes, nuclei, cytoplasm, and cell walls) up to tissues, organs, and the whole plant itself, and on up to entire communities (like forests, grassland, crops, and landscapes). The biological functions that are being studied from biomechanical and mechanobiological perspectives cover most of the physiological functions of plants—growth, sensing, morphogenesis, differentiation, water relations, sap flow and osmoregulation, support and posture control, above- and below-ground exploration, mating and seed dispersal, acclimation, and resistance to wind and currents and to drought, gravity, pathogens, and herbivory.

Sports Biomechanics

Biomechanics in Sport incorporates detailed analysis of sport movements in order to minimize the risk of injury and improve sports performance. Sport and Exercise Biomechanics encompasses the area of science concerned with the analysis of the mechanics of human movement. It refers to the description, detailed analysis and assessment of human movement during sport activities. Mechanics is a branch of physics that is concerned with the description of motion/movement and how forces create motion/movement. In other words sport biomechanics is the science of explaining how and why the human body moves in the way that it does. In sport and exercise that definition is often extended to also consider the interaction between the performer and their equipment and environment.

Newton's Laws of Motion

Newton's Three Laws of Motion explain how forces create motion in sport. These laws are usually referred to as the Laws of Inertia, Acceleration, and Reaction.

1. Law of Inertia - Newton's First Law of inertia states that objects tend to resist changes in their state of motion. An object in motion will tend to stay in motion and an object at rest will tend to stay at rest unless acted upon by a force. *Example* - The body of a player quickly sprinting down the field will tend to want to retain that motion unless muscular forces can overcome this inertia.

2. Law of Acceleration - Newton's Second Law precisely explains how much motion a force creates. The acceleration (tendency of an object to change speed or direction) an object experiences is proportional to the size of the force and inversely proportional to the object's mass ($F = ma$). *Example* - If a player improves leg strength through training while maintaining the same body mass, they will have an increased ability to accelerate the body using the legs, resulting in better agility and speed. This also relates to the ability to rotate segments.

3. Law of Reaction - The Third Law states that for every action (force) there is an equal and opposite reaction force. This means that forces do not act alone, but occur in equal and opposite pairs between interacting bodies. Example - The force created by the legs "pushing" against the ground results in ground reaction forces in which the ground "pushes back" and allows the player to move across the court (As the Earth is much more massive than the player, the player accelerates and moves rapidly, while the Earth does not really accelerate or move at all). This action-reaction also occurs at impact with the ball as the force applied to the ball is matched with an equal and opposite force applied to the racket/body.

Momentum

Newton' Second Law is also related to the variable momentum, which is the product of an object's velocity and mass. Momentum is essentially the quantity of motion an object possesses. Momentum can be transferred from one object to another. There are different types of momentum which each have a different impact on the sport.

- Linear Momentum, which is momentum in a straight line. Example - Linear momentum is created as the athlete sprints in a straight line down the 100m straight on the track.

- Angular Momentum, which is rotational momentum and is created by the rotations of the various body segments e.g. the open stance forehand uses significant angular momentum. The tremendous increase in the use of angular momentum in groundstrokes and serves has had a significant impact on the game of tennis. One of the main reasons for the increase in power of the game today is the incorporation of angular momentum into groundstroke and serves techniques. In tennis, the angular momentum developed by the coordinated action of body segments transfers to the linear momentum of the racket at impact

Center of Gravity

The Center of Gravity (COG) is an imaginary point around which body weight is evenly distributed the center of gravity of the human body can change considerably because the segments of the body can move their masses with joint rotations. This concept is critical to understanding balance and stability and how gravity affects sport techniques.

The direction of the force of gravity through the body is downward, towards the center of the earth and through the COG. This line of gravity is important to understand and visualize when determining a person's ability to successfully maintain Balance. When the line of gravity falls outside the Base of Support (BOS), then a reaction is needed in order to stay balanced.

The center of gravity of a squash racket is a far simpler process and can usually be found by identifying the point where the racket balances on your finger or another narrow object.

Balance

Balance is the ability of a player to control their equilibrium or stability. You need to have a good understanding of both static and dynamic balance:

- Static Balance - The ability to control the body while the body is stationary. It is the ability to maintain the body in some fixed posture. Static balance is the ability to maintain postural stability and orientation with center of mass over the base of support and body at rest.

- Dynamic Balance - The ability to control the body during motion. Defining dynamic postural stability is more challenging, Dynamic balance is the ability to transfer the vertical projection of the center of gravity around the supporting base of support. Dynamic balance is the ability to maintain postural stability and orientation with center of mass over the base of support while the body parts are in motion.

Lower Limb Biomechanics

As humans ambulation is our main form of movement that is we walk upright and are very reliant on our legs to move us about. How the foot strikes the ground and the knock on effect this has up the lower limbs to the knee, hips, pelvis and low back in particular has become a subject of much debate and controversy in recent years.

Lower limb biomechanics refers to a complex interplay between the joints, muscles and nervous system which results in a certain patterning of movement, often referred to as 'alignment'. Much of the debate centres around what is considered 'normal' and what is considered 'abnormal' in biomechanical terms as well as the extent to which we should intervene should abnormal findings be found on assessment.

Foot & Ankle Biomechanics

The foot and ankle form a complex system which consists of 26 bones, 33 joints and more than 100 muscles, tendons and ligaments. It functions as a rigid structure for weight bearing and it can also function as a flexible structure to conform to uneven terrain. The foot and ankle provide various important functions which include: supporting body weight, providing balance, shock absorption, transferring ground reaction forces, compensating for proximal malalignment, and substituting hand function in individuals with upper extremity amputation/paralysis all which are key when involved with any exercise or sport involving the lower limbs. This page examines in detail the biomechanics of the foot and ankle and its role in locomotion.

Q Angle

An understanding of the normal anatomical and biomechanical features of the patellofemoral joint is essential to any evaluation of knee function. The Q angle formed by the vector for the combined pull of the quadriceps femoris muscle and the patellar tendon, is important because of the lateral pull it exerts on the patella.

The direction and magnitude of force produced by the quadriceps muscle has great influence on patellofemoral joint biomechanics. The line of force exerted by the quadriceps is lateral to the joint line mainly due to large cross-sectional area and force potential of the vastus lateralis. Since there exists an association between patellofemoral pathology and excessive lateral tracking of the patella, assessing the overall lateral line of pull of the quadriceps relative to the patella is a meaningful clinical measure. Such a measure is referred to as the Quadriceps angle or Q angle. It was initially described by Brattstrom.

Biomechanics of Gait

Sandra J. Shultz describes gait as: "someone's manner of ambulation or locomotion, involves the total body. Gait speed determines the contribution of each body segment. Normal walking speed primarily involves the lower extremities, with the arms and trunk providing stability and balance. The faster the speed, the more the body depends on the upper extremities and trunk for propulsion as well as balance and stability. The legs continue to do the most work as the joints produce greater ranges of motion trough greater muscle responses. In the bipedal system the three major joints of the lower body and pelvis work with each other as muscles and momentum move the body forward. The degree to which the body's center of gravity moves during forward translation defines efficiency. The body's center moves both side to side and up and down during gait." Bipedal walking is an important characteristic of humans. This page will present information about the different phases of the gait cycle and important functions of the foot while walking.

Upper Limb Biomechanics

Correct biomechanics are as important in upper limb activities as they are in lower limb activities. The capabilities of the upper extremity are varied and impressive. With the same basic anatomical structure of the arm, forearm, hand, and fingers, major league Baseball Pitchers pitch fastballs at 40 m/s, Swimmers cross the English Channel, Gymnasts perform the iron cross, and Olympic Boxers in weight classes ranging from flyweight to super heavyweight showed a range of 447 to 1,066 pounds of peak punching force.

The structure of the upper extremity is composed of the shoulder girdle and the upper limb. The shoulder girdle consists of the scapula and clavicle, and the upper limb is composed of the arm, forearm, wrist, hand, and fingers. However, a kinematic chain extends from the cervical and upper thoracic spine to the fingertips. Only when certain multiple segments are completely fixed can these parts possibly function independently in mechanical roles.

Scapulohumeral Rhythm

Scapulohumeral rhythm (also referred to as glenohumeral rhythm) is the kinematic interaction between the scapula and the humerus, first published by Codman in the 1930s. This interaction is important for the optimal function of the shoulder. When there is a change of the normal position of the scapula) relative to the humerus, can this can cause a disfunction of the scapulohumeral rhythm. The change of the normal position is also called scapular dyskinesia. Various studies of the mechanism of the shoulder joint have attempted to describe the global motion capacity of the shoulder refer to that description, can you evaluate the shoulder to see if the function is correct? And explain the complex interactions between components involved in placing the hand in space.

Running Biomechanics

Running is similar to walking in terms of locomotor activity. However, there are key differences. Having the ability to walk does not mean that the individual has the ability to run . There are some differences between the gait and run cycle - the gait cycle is one third longer in time, the ground reaction force is smaller in the gait cycle (so the load is lower), and the velocity is much higher. In running, there is also just one stance phase while in stepping there are two. Shock absorption is also much larger in comparison to walking. This explains why runners have more overload injuries .

Running Requires:

- Greater Balance

- Greater Muscle Strength

- Greater Joint Range of Movement

Cycling Biomechanics

Cycling was initially invented by Baron Carl von Drais in 1817, but not as we know it. This was a machine which initially had two wheels that were connected by a wooden plank with a rudder device for steering. It involved people running along the ground whilst sitting down; giving them the name of a 'running machine' or a velocipied. This was solely used by the male population at the time of invention. The velocipied then made a huge design development in the 1860's at the Michaux factory in Paris. They added leaver arms to the front wheel which were propelled by pedals at the feet. This was the first conventional bicycle, and since then and up until the current day the bicycle has made great design and technological advances. A survey in 2014 estimated that over 43% of the United Kingdom population have or have access to a bike and 8% of the population aged 5 and above cycled 3 or more times a week. With such a large amount of people cycling, whether it be professional, recreational or for commuting this increase the chance of developing an injury, so it is time we understood the biomechanics of cycling.

Baseball Pitching Biomechanics

Baseball pitching is one of the most intensely studying athletic motion. Although focus has been more on shoulder, entire body movement is required to perform a baseball pitching. Throwing is also considered one of the fastest human motions performed, and maximum humeral internal rotation velocity reaches about 7000 to 75000/second.

Tennis Biomechanics

Tennis biomechanics is a very complex task. Consider hitting a tennis ball. First the athlete needs to see the ball coming off their opponent's racquet. Then, in order, they have to judge the speed, spin, trajectory and, most importantly, the direction of the tennis ball. The player then needs to adjust their body position quickly to move around the ball. As the player returns prepares to hit the ball the body is in motion, the ball is moving both in a linear and rotation direction if there is pin on the ball, and the racquet is also in motion. The player must coordinate all these movements in approximately a half a second so they strike the ball as close to the center of the racquet in order to produce the desired spin, speed and direction for return of the ball. A mistake in any of these movements can create an error.

Nanobiomechanics

Nanobiomechanics, also called nanoscale biomechanics, is a field of biomedical technology that involves measurement of the mechanical characteristics of individual living cells. This is done using instruments that can produce, detect, and measure forces on the order of a few piconewtons (trillionths of a newton , where a trillionth is equal to

0.000000000001 or 10^{-12}). Nanobiomechanics is part of the larger field of nanoscale biomedical research.

One of the most significant potential applications of nanobiomechanics is the diagnosis of, and the development of new treatments for, disease conditions. In humans and animals, physiological disorders are correlated with specific changes in individual cells. An example is malaria, a disease that affects millions of people, particularly in the tropics. While malaria can be treated, a completely effective vaccine or cure in humans has not yet been found. In people who have malaria, the red blood cells lose much of their flexibility. Using nanobiomechanics, researchers have been able to measure the extent to which this loss of flexibility occurs. Knowing the ways in which disease conditions affect cells may lead to new ways of treating diseases that have heretofore defied resolution.

The mechanical properties of living cells can affect their physical interactions with their surrounding extracellular matrix, potentially influencing the process of mechanical signal transduction in living tissues. Alterations in cell properties are of fundamental importance for a wide range of processes, and changes in cell mechanics are associated with conditions such as osteoarthritis, asthma, cancer, inflammation and malaria. The mechanical properties of living cells have been quantified using various testing methods, such as micropipette aspiration, magnetic twisting cytometry, optical tweezers and nanoindentation. From the perspective of cell mechanics, one should be aware of what is measured with respect to particular techniques. For example, it is often observed that the cell appears softer during micropipette aspirations compared with cytocompression or indentation with a large spherical tip. During micropipette aspirations, it was observed that the cytoskeleton can be disrupted. In such a case, there is no (or very limited) tensile stress in the actin fibres, which significantly contributes to cell stiffness. Therefore, cell mechanics can be approximated, as cytosol reinforced with bundles of actin fibres (with diameter of 9–10 nm). The weight concentration of actin fibres is 1–10% for non-muscle cells and 10–20% for muscle cells, and the elastic modulus of these actin fibres is 1.3–2.5 GPa .

Cells would sense and respond to the nanoscale (or microscale) features on the materials surface. For example, when in contact with implanted devices or scaffold materials, cells interact with nanoscale (or submicroscale) surface features in topography and surface chemistry. Therefore, the nanobiomechanics of the living cells is very important for surface design of the implanted materials and the scaffold materials for tissue engineering. In addition, it also helps us to improve the understanding of cell interaction with nanoparticles, which is important for nanotoxicology and nanomedicine. Compared with other measurement techniques, nanoindentation has the advantage of *in situ* imaging of the indented cells with a high resolution, a very good control of the probe position and loading (or unloading) speed, and the flexibility of using different probe geometries (e.g. flat punch spherical, pyramidal and conical). It also has the unique feature of mapping the measured mechanical properties over the investigated surface of the sample. However, data interpretation for nanoindentation of living cells is often difficult.

Therefore, the goals of this study were (i) to present the strategy of selecting the right type of indenter tips; (ii) to illustrate cell mechanics at different test conditions; (iii) to discuss the mechanical models that enable extracting the mechanical properties of living cells during nanoindentation.

Experimental Aspects

Nanoindenter Apparatus and Atomic Force Microscope

Nanoindentation is also known as depth sensing indentation, in which the indentation load–depth–time $(P - \delta - t)$ profile is recorded. It enables probing the mechanical properties at the nanoscale or microscale. For such a small-scale indentation, there are different approaches to take with respect to the testing instrumentation. In general, we could divide them into nanoindenter apparatus and atomic force microscope (AFM). The key difference between the commercial nanoindentation apparatus and the AFM is on the different transducer operation mechanisms: the former uses electrical capacitance gages or magnetic coils to directly drive the indenter into the sample. When a voltage is applied, an electrostatic force is generated between the pick-up electrode and drive plates, resulting in the movement of the pick-up electrode between the drive plates. While the AFM actuates the tip indirectly via the bending of a cantilever, the AFM operates by measuring attractive or repulsive forces between a tip and the sample, which causes vertical deflection of the cantilever. To detect the displacement of the cantilever, a laser is reflected at the back of the cantilever and collected in a photodiode.

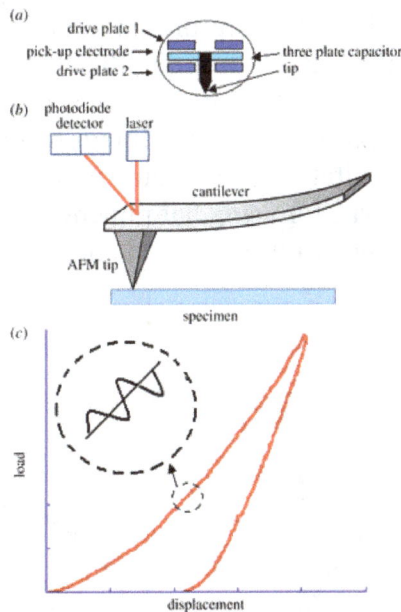

Figure (*a*) Schematic of electrical capacitance gages that drives nanoindenter, (*b*) the bending of a cantilever that actuates the AFM tip and (*c*) dynamic drive signal superposed with the force curve which enables dynamic mechanical measurement during nanoindentation. (Online version in colour.)

In addition to quasi-static loading, a dynamic drive signal can be superposed with the force curve in both the nanoindenter apparatus and the AFM . This enables measurement of the storage modulus, loss modulus and phase angle, which can be converted to the instantaneous modulus, equilibrium modulus and viscosity.

The nanoindenter apparatus allows better control of the indentation force and displacement. The AFM offers the unique advantages of applying very small indentation forces (below 100 pN), but accurate calibration is not easy. Owing to ultra-high resolutions in force and displacement, AFM nanoindentation is particularly useful for probing living cells and subcellular components such as the cell membrane and cytoskeleton.

Choice of Appropriate Atomic Force Microscope Tips

There are various tip geometries that can be fitted with the AFM cantilever for nanoindentation tests. The advantages and disadvantages of these tips are discussed as follows. The shape of cells can be spherical or spreading in morphology, depending on the physiological conditions and microenvironment of the living cells and cell types. The choice of appropriate AFM tips depends on cell morphology, cell type and what is of interest (cellular mechanics or subcellular mechanics).

Flat Punch

Indentation of cells with a flat-ended cylindrical punch (figure) is also known as cytoindentation . In this case, the size of the flat punch is much smaller than the cell. This type of indenter is preferred for a very soft and fragile cellular or subcellular structure. The advantage is that data interpretation is relatively straightforward because it avoids the complication of determining the contact area. The contact area is less likely to be affected by thermal drift or creep. The drawback is the spatial resolution is relatively limited compared with the pointed indenter (e.g. pyramid and conical tip); therefore, it is not suitable to characterize fine features. In addition, there are also other practical concerns for using flat punches, such as alignment, detection of contact point and force concentration around edges. The tips are usually made of silicon or glass.

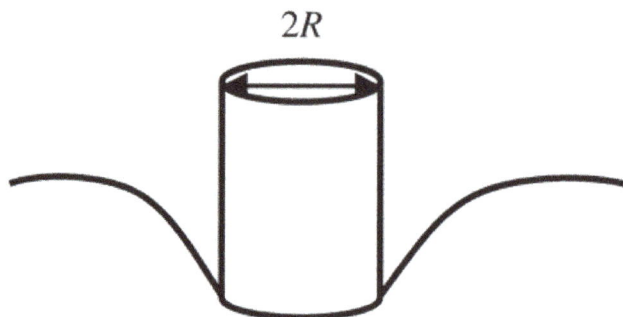

Figure: Schematic of nanoindentation by a flat-ended cylindrical punch.

Spherical Tip

This type of indenter is also ideal for very soft and fragile cellular or subcellular structures. This type of tip would be particularly useful if the elastic properties of the materials were to change with strain. As the effective strain is related to the ratio of the contact radius and the tip radius, it enables determining the stress–strain curves of the indented materials. The typical spherical tip is made of glass which is easy to manufacture. Similar to the flat punch probe, the spherical glass probe is less likely to cause damage to cells . Again, this may not be good for probing fine features. The typical radius of the probe for indentation of cells is 2.5–10 µm. The representative strain for the spherical tip is the ratio of the contact radius over the effective tip radius.

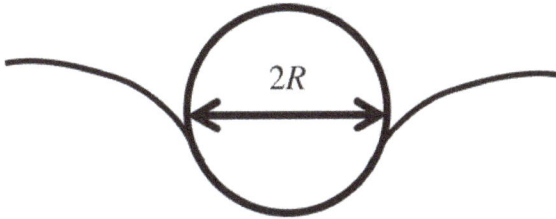

Figure: Schematic of nanoindentation by a spherical tip.

Pyramid Tip

At a given penetration, the pyramid indenter yields a much smaller contact area compared with the spherical and flat punch tips. It is particularly useful to probe fine features such as the cytoskeleton. Owing to the crystalline structure of silicon, it can be easily etched at certain plane directions, enabling massive production of the probes. The drawback is that the sharp edges may damage the fragile cell membrane or nuclear membrane; therefore, it is not recommended for indentation of living cells.

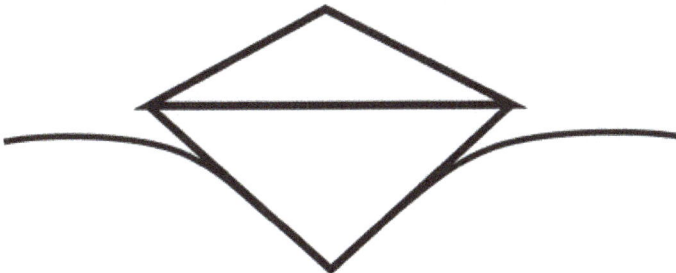

Figure: Schematic of nanoindentation by a pyramid tip.

Conical Tip

Similar to the pyramid tip, the conical tip yields a much smaller contact area compared with the spherical and flat punch tip. Compared with the pyramid tip, it is less likely to cause damage in lateral directions because it does not have sharp edges. It also circumvents complicated data interpretation owing to coupling of anisotropic soft materials and orientation of the pyramid tip. In principle, the semi-included angle of the probe will not affect the measured elastic or plastic properties, if the appropriate models are used. But it affects the relationship between the yield strength and hardness. At a given penetration, the deformation-affected volume is related to the semi-included angle of the probe. Therefore, to eliminate the effect of the substrate or the surrounding matrix, one may need to choose a tip with smaller semi-included angle although the increased stress intensity underneath the very sharp tip might cause puncture of the cell membrane. But this influence is not that significant if the tip radius is much smaller than the penetration. When using this probe to do indentation at shallow penetration, it would only sense localized properties mainly resulting from the cell membrane with the underlying cortex or individual cytoskeleton. Sometimes, it may simply measure the bending stiffness of the cell membrane. In such a case, it is unlikely to obtain the mechanical properties of the whole cell. For similar geometries such as a cone (a cylindrical punch can be treated as cone with a semi-apical angle of 90°) and a pyramid, the effective strain is a constant and related to the semi-apical angle (θ).

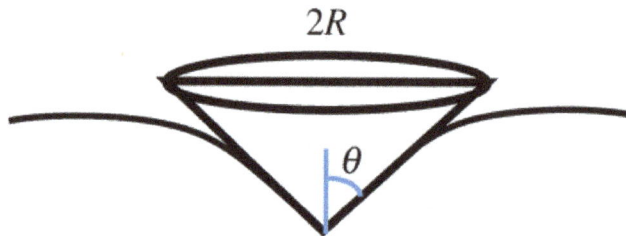

Figure: Schematic of nanoindentation by a conical tip.

Extended Atomic Force Microscope Testing Rigs

In recent years, another type of indentation, cytocompression, has been widely used to assess the mechanical properties of single cells. In principle, this is an extended AFM indentation on top of cytoindentation. The primary difference in the deformation mechanisms for cytoindentation and cytocompression is in the relative size between the flat punch and the cell. The former has a flat punch diameter well below that of cell. The latter has a flat punch diameter exceeding that of the cell. In such a case, data interpretation is the same as in normal compression tests. The indenter (i.e. the flat plate) is often made of glass, which enables *in situ* observation of cell deformation.

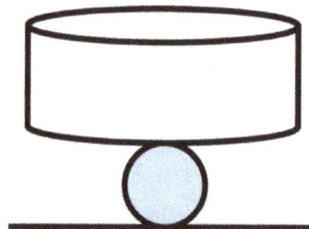

Figure: Schematic of cytocompression of a spherical cell.

Mechanical Modelling

Estimation of cell mechanics requires the use of analytical models (or empirical models) of which there are two principal types, namely structure-based models and continuum models. The former include tensegrity and percolation models, which consider cell mechanics to be dominant by the collective discrete loading bearing element. The latter include linear elastic, hyperelastic, poroelastic (also known as biphasic model) and viscoelastic models. The continuum model may be interpreted as load-bearing elements that are infinitesimally small relative to the size of the cell.

Structure-based Models

Tensegrity model

The tensegrity model is based on the use of isolated components under compression inside a net of continuous tension, in such a way that the compressed members do not touch each other and the pre-stressed, tensioned cables, as shown in. This model was coined by Buckminster Fuller in the 1960s. Such a concept was then introduced by Ingber to cell mechanics. It assumes that a cell stabilizes its structure by incorporating compression-resistant elements to resist the global pull of the contractile cytoskeleton. This simple stick and string tensegrity model predicts that a cell appears round when unattached (owing to the internal tension) or attached with a very soft substrate, and spreads out when attached to a stiff substrate. All these agree well with experimental observations.

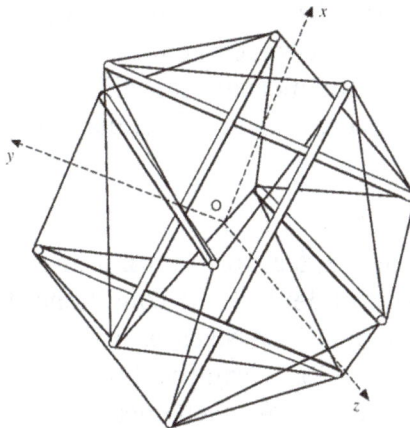

Figure: A schematic tensegrity model of cell structure for a spherical cell.

Percolation Models

The percolation theory describes the behaviour of connected clusters in a random manner. It was introduced in mathematics and then it was applied to materials science. Recently, such a theory was introduced to describe the cell structure and its mechanics. The percolation cluster contains substructures of tensegrity on a small scale. These tensegrity substructures are likely to contribute to inherent tension in the cytoskeleton. Owing to the random nature of their interconnection, percolation networks are so flexible that they can easily adapt to the dynamic conditions that affect cells.

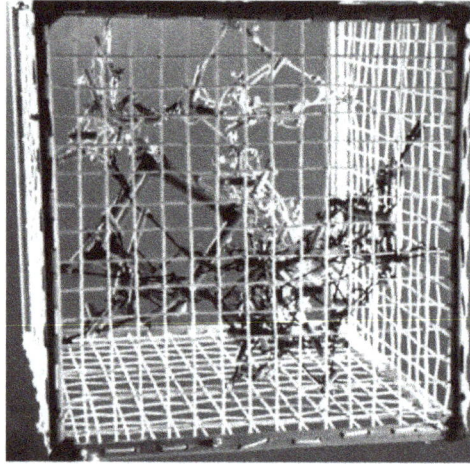

Figure: A schematic percolation model of cell structure. The smaller interior cube representing the nucleus is supported by the pre-stressed cytoskeletal network.

Summary of Structure-based Models

The percolation and tensegrity models of the cytoskeleton are not mutually exclusive, but complementary. As commented in, it is possible that during evolution certain locally ordered tensegrity-type structures may have emerged from more randomly interconnected percolation structures. These structure-based models are very successful at explaining a range of physical observations on cell mechanics such as cell spreading, cell migration, cell detachment and mechanosensation, etc. But it is difficult to quantify the mechanical properties of living cells or subcellular structures.

Continuum Models

Despite neglecting microstructural features, continuum models enable quantifying the mechanical properties of cells under various conditions that could provide essential information of cellular subpopulations disease, malignant transformation and cell–materials interactions. However, it is worth pointing out that there is no universal mechanical model available to quantify the mechanical properties of living cells at various physiological and microenvironmental conditions, because living cells can dynamically adapt to their environment. The feasible methodology is to choose appropriate models according to testing condition for a given cell type.

Elastic Model

If the tests were performed slowly such that the cell reaches equilibrium, then it is reasonable to use elastic models. At relatively small deformation, a simple linear elastic model may be used to find the Young modulus of the cell (E). Evidence has been shown that this simple elastic model can still reveal useful insights of cell mechanics such as the stiffness ratio of the nucleus over the cytoplasm.

If the cell undergoes large deformation, then it may reach the nonlinear elastic region. The neo-Hookean (NH) model, also known as the Gaussian model, is one of the most widely used nonlinear elastic (or hyperelastic) models owing to its simplicity. For example, it has been successfully used to model the deformation of single cells in cytocompression tests. For incompressible materials, the NH model has the following energy function:

$$W = C_1\left(\lambda_1^2 + \lambda_2^2 + \lambda_3^2 - 3\right),$$

Where W is the strain energy density, $l_j(j = 1,2,3)$ are the three principal stretch ratios. The Young modulus E is given by

$$E = 6C_1.$$

Other more sophisticated hyperealstic models have also been developed, such as the polynominal and Ogden models. The strain energy function for the former is given by the flowing equation:

$$W = \sum_{i+j=1}^{N} C_{ij}\left(\lambda_1^2 + \lambda_2^2 + \lambda_3^2 - 3\right)^i \left(\frac{1}{\lambda_1^2} + \frac{1}{\lambda_2^2} + \frac{1}{\lambda_3^2} - 3\right)^j.$$

The Young modulus E is given by

$$E = 6\left(C_{10} + C_{01}\right).$$

The Ogden model can describe a wide range of strain-hardening characteristics, and it takes the following form as described in previous studies:

$$W = \sum_{i=1}^{n} \frac{2\mu_i}{\alpha_i^2}\left(\lambda_1^{\alpha_i} + \lambda_2^{\alpha_i} + \lambda_3^{\alpha_i} - 3\right),$$

Where α_i is strain-hardening exponent. The constants μ_i are related to the initial Young modulus E, by

$$E = 3\sum_{i=1}^{n} \mu_i$$

This model has been adopted to describe cell mechanics when the chondrocyte is embedded in various hydrogel scaffolds.

Poroelastic Model

The poroelastic model attributes the time-dependence to the flow of a fluid through an elastic (or viscoelastic) porous solid. Such a model was first proposed by Biot and was based on the assumptions of linearity between the stress (s_{ij}, p) and the strain (ε_{ij}, ρ) and reversibility of the deformation process. With the respective addition of the scalar quantities p and ρ to the stress and strain group, the linear constitutive relations can be obtained by extending the known elastic expressions. The most general form for isotropic material constitutive behaviour response is described as follows:

$$\varepsilon_{ij} = \frac{\sigma_{ij}}{2G} - \left(\frac{1}{6G} - \frac{1}{9k}\right)\delta_{ij}\sigma_{kk} + \frac{\delta_{ij}p}{3H}$$

And

$$\rho = \frac{\sigma_{kk}}{3H} + \frac{p}{M},$$

where K and G are bulk and shear modulus of the drained elastic solid. The parameters H and M characterize the coupling between solid and fluid stress and strain.

This model was originally developed for soil mechanics and it was then applied to describe the mechanics of hydrogels and tissues such as bone and cartilage. Very recently, it has also been applied to cell mechanics. When it comes down to cell mechanics, the material properties of interest include the shear modulus G (or aggregate modulus H_A), and Poisson's ratio of the solid matrix and Darcy permeability k. The permeability could be analogous to the diffusion coefficient, but driven by the mechanical gradient instead of the chemical gradient.

During stress relaxation, it gives

$$\frac{P(t) - P(\infty)}{P(0) - P(\infty)} = g(\tau),$$

Where $P(\infty)$ and $P(0)$ signify the force at infinite time $(t=\infty)$ and $t= 0$, respectively.

Where the normalized time τ is given by

$$\tau = \frac{Dt}{a^2}$$

Where a is the contact radius and t is time.

The diffusivity D is given by

$$D = \frac{2(1-v)}{1-2v}\frac{Gk}{\eta},$$

Where v, G, k and η are Poisson's ratio, shear modulus and permeability of the solid matrix and viscosity of the solvent, respectively.

The equilibrium Young modulus E is given by

$$E = 2G(1+v)$$

The relation between the aggregate modulus and the Young modulus is given by

$$H_A = \frac{E(1-v)}{(1+v)(1-2v)}.$$

This poroelastic model is quite similar to the biphasic theory of the mixture of an incompressible solid and incompressible fluid which was independently developed by Mow and Bowen . In addition, by replacing the elastic media with viscoelastic media to account for the intrinsic viscoelastic properties of the actin filaments, a more complex model can be used to describe soft tissue or cell mechanics. When the cell is exposed to an ionic solution, the ionic charge also contributes to the mechanical responses of cells. In such a case, a third phase (i.e. the ionic phase) can be included in the constitutive equation, which is called the triphasic model.

Spring-dashpot Viscoelastic Models

The basic premise of viscoelasticity of this type is that it replaces some elastic springs with a time-dependent dashpot. These spring-dashpot models usually refer to viscoelastic models. In a general manner, the empirical Prony series has been used to describe the material's time-dependent constitutive response in the experimental time domain.

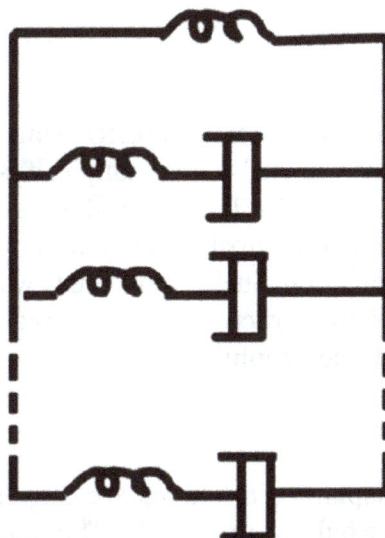

Figure: Schematic of the generalized Maxwell model.

For stress relaxation, the relaxation shear modulus $G(t)$ in an empirical Prony series is given by

$$G(t) = G_\infty + \sum G_i \exp\left(-\frac{t}{\tau_i}\right),$$

Where G_∞ is the equilibrium shear modulus and the instantaneous shear modulus $G_0 = G_\infty + \sum G_i$ or creep, the creep compliance $J(t)$ in an empirical Prony series is given by

$$J(t) \, C_0 - \sum C_i \exp\left(-\frac{t}{\tau_i}\right),$$

Where the parameters C_i are associated with compliance values (inverse shear modulus).

The stress relaxation modulus and the creep compliance are not explicitly inverse in the time domain but are in the Laplace domain (i.e. $G(s)J(s) = s^2$).

The equilibrium shear modulus (G_∞) and the instantaneous shear modulus (G_0) can be determined by the following equations:

$$G_\infty = \frac{1}{C_0}$$

And

$$G_0 = \frac{1}{C_0 - \sum C_i}$$

Power-law Rheology

Power-law rheology ($G(t) \approx t^{-n}$, where n is a positive constant) has also been adopted to describe the mechanics of certain cells. For example, it is found that $n = 0.2$ for lung epithelial cells during stress relaxation. The physical basis of this power law may be related to molecular adjustment of the cytoskeleton matrix, which is similar to soft glassy materials close to the glass transition. Such a model may work better for those cells that do not have a strong cytoskeleton structure. For example, such a power-law rheology model has also been applied to neutrophils and macrophages.

Nanoindentation Models

Once the AFM deflection–displacement curves are converted to force–displacement curves, indentation theories would be applicable. The models below are based on assumptions of small deformation and negligible tip–cell adhesions.

Elastic Nanoindentation Models

Flat punch: the force–displacement ($P - \delta$) relation is given by

$$P = \frac{4GR}{(1-v)}\delta,$$

Where R and v are the radius of the flat punch and Poisson's ratio, respectively.

Spherical tip: the force–displacement relation is given by the Hertz elastic model

$$P = \frac{8}{3}\frac{G}{1-v}\sqrt{R}\delta^{3/2},$$

Where R are the radius of the spherical indenter.

Conical tip: the force–displacement relation is given by

$$P = \frac{4G\tan\theta}{\pi(1-v)}\delta^2,$$

Where θ is the semi-included angle of the conical indenter.

Poroelastic–nanoindentation Models

Flat punch: the force–time ($P - t$) relation is given by

$$P(0) = 8G\delta a$$

and

$$g(\tau)\frac{P(t) - P(\infty)}{P(0) - P(\infty)}$$
$$= 1.304\exp\left(-\sqrt{\tau}\right) - 0.304\exp(-0.254\tau).$$

Spherical tip: the force–time relation is given by

$$P(0) = \frac{16}{3}G\delta a,$$

and

$$g(\tau) = 0.491\exp\left(-0.908\sqrt{\tau}\right) + 0.509\exp\left(-1.679\tau\right).$$

Conical tip: the force–time relation is given by

$$P(0) = 4G\delta a,$$

And

$$g(\tau) = 0.493 = \exp\left(-0.822\sqrt{\tau}\right) + 0.507\exp\left(-1.348\tau\right),$$

Where a is the contact radius, and τ is the normalized time constant as defined earlier.

A simpler poroelastic model to describe cell mechanics has been presented in, which considers fluid propagates through a cell owing to a local pressure increase in a two-dimensional manner. This model requires other techniques to determine the pore size and viscosity, rather than relying on the analysis of the force–time–displacement curve alone. For pore size, it can be estimated by hindered tracer particle diffusion experiments, and for viscosity it can be estimated by a nanoparticle diffusion experiment.

Viscoelastic-nanoindentation Models

When viscoelastic models were adopted, experimentalists used either the stress relaxation (for tests performed under displacement control) or creep (for tests performed under force control) period to determine viscoelastic parameters. It is advantageous to use stress relaxation or creep for data analysis because they circumvent the possible complexity in nonlinear changes during ramping.

Flat punch: the following force–time and the displacement–time relations can be obtained by incorporating the viscoelastic model into equation $G_\infty = \dfrac{1}{C_0}$

Stress relaxation

$$P(t) = \frac{4R}{3(1-v)} \int_0^t G(t-\tau)\delta(\tau)\frac{d\delta(\tau)}{d\tau}\,d\tau,$$

and

$$\text{Creep}: \delta^{3/2}(t) = \frac{3(1-v)}{8\sqrt{R}} \int_0^t J(t-r)\frac{dp(\tau)}{d\tau}\,d\tau.$$

More rigorous analytical solutions were given by, which consider that the elastic components may have different Poisson's ratios.

Spherical tip: the force–time and the displacement–time relations are given by

Stress relaxation :

$$P(t) = \frac{8\sqrt{R}}{3(1-v)} \int\limits_0^t G(t-\tau) \frac{d\delta^{3/2}(\tau)}{d\tau} d\tau,$$

Creep : $\delta^{3/2}(t) = \frac{3(1-v)}{8\sqrt{R}} \int\limits_0^t J(t-r) \frac{dp(\tau)}{d\tau} d\tau.$

Conical tip: the force–time and the displacement–time relations are given by [

$$P(t) = \frac{4\tan\theta}{\pi(1-v)} \int\limits_0^t G(t-\tau)\delta(\tau) \frac{d\delta(\tau)}{d\tau} d\tau,$$

and

$$\text{Creep}: \delta^2(t) = \frac{\pi(1-v)}{4\tan\theta} \int\limits_0^t J(t-\tau) \frac{dP(\tau)}{d\tau} d\tau.$$

For complicated load–time or displacement–time histories, Boltzmann hereditary integrals can be used to find full $P - \delta - t$ profiles.

References

- Dynamics-physics, science: britannica.com, Retrieved 24 June 2018
- What-are-the-applications-of-dynamics-in-biomedical-engineering: quora.com, Retrieved 19 July 2018
- Biomechanics-definitions-4: strengthandconditioningresearch.com, Retrieved 15 May 2018
- Biomechanics-In-Sport: physio-pedia.com, Retrieved 12 March 2018
- Nanobiomechanics-nanoscale-biomechanics: techtarget.com, Retrieved 31 March 2018

4

Biomaterials

Any substance, which is engineered to interact with biological systems for therapeutic or diagnostic purposes, is called a biomaterial. The study of biomaterials is under the discipline of biomaterials science or biomaterials engineering. An understanding of biomaterials is facilitated by a study of biocompatibility, nanocellulose, cell encapsulation, etc. which have been extensively discussed in this chapter.

Biomaterials plays an integral role in medicine today—restoring function and facilitating healing for people after injury or disease. Biomaterials may be natural or synthetic and are used in medical applications to support, enhance, or replace damaged tissue or a biological function. The first historical use of biomaterials dates to antiquity, when ancient Egyptians used sutures made from animal sinew. The modern field of biomaterials combines medicine, biology, physics, and chemistry, and more recent influences from tissue engineering and materials science. The field has grown significantly in the past decade due to discoveries in tissue engineering, regenerative medicine, and more.

Metals, ceramics, plastic, glass, and even living cells and tissue all can be used in creating a biomaterial. They can be reengineered into molded or machined parts, coatings, fibers, films, foams, and fabrics for use in biomedical products and devices. These may include heart valves, hip joint replacements, dental implants, or contact lenses. They often are biodegradable, and some are bio-absorbable, meaning they are eliminated gradually from the body after fulfilling a function.

Polymers

There are a large number of polymeric materials that have been used as implants or part of implant systems. The polymeric systems include acrylics, polyamides, polyesters, polyethylene, polysiloxanes, polyurethane, and a number of reprocessed biological materials.

Some of the applications include the use of membranes of ethylene-vinyl-acetate (EVA) copolymer for controlled release and the use of poly-glycolic acid for use as a resorbable suture material. Some other typical biomedical polymeric materials applications include: artificial heart, kidney, liver, pancreas, bladder, bone cement, catheters, contact lenses, cornea and eye-lens replacements, external and internal ear repairs, heart valves, cardiac assist devices, implantable pumps, joint replacements, pacemaker, encapsulations, soft-tissue replacement, artificial blood vessels, artificial skin, and sutures.

As bioengineers search for designs of ever increasing capabilities to meet the needs of medical practice, polymeric materials alone and in combination with metals and ceramics are becoming increasingly incorporated into devices used in the body.

Metals

The metallic systems most frequently used in the body are:

(a) Iron-base alloys of the 316L stainless steel

(b) Titanium and titanium-base alloys, such as

    (i) Ti- 6% Al- 4% V, and commercially pure 98.9%

    (ii) $Ti - Ni$ $(55\% \ Ni$ and $45\% \ Ti)$

(c) Cobalt base alloys of four types

    (i) Cr $(27$-$30\%)$, Mo $(5$-$7\%)$, Ni $(2$-$5\%)$

    (ii) Cr $(19$-$21\%)$, Ni $(9$-$11\%)$, W $(14$-$16\%)$

    (iii) Cr $(18$-$22\%)$, Fe $(4$-$6\%)$, Ni $(15$-$25\%)$, W $(3$-$4\%)$

    (iv) Cr $(19$-$20\%)$, Mo $(9$-$10\%)$, Ni $(33$-$37\%)$

The most commonly used implant metals are the 316L stainless steels, Ti-6%-4%V, and Cobalt base alloys of type "i" and "ii". Other metal systems being investigated include Cobalt-base alloys of type "iii" and "iv", and Niobium and shape memory alloys, of which (Ti 45% - 55%Ni) is receiving most attention.

Composite Materials

Composite materials have been extensively used in dentistry and prosthesis designers are now incorporating these materials into other applications. Typically, a matrix of ultrahigh-molecular-weight polyethylene (UHMWPE) is reinforced with carbon fibers. These carbon fibers are made by pyrolizing acrylic fibers to obtain oriented graphitic structure of high tensile strength and high modulus of elasticity. The carbon fibers are 6- 15mm in diameter, and they are randomly oriented in the matrix. In order for the high modulus property of the reinforcing fibers to strengthen the matrix, a sufficient interfacial bond between the fiber and matrix must be achieved during the manufacturing process. This fiber reinforced composite can then be used to make a variety of implants such as intra-medullary rods and artificial joints. Since the mechanical properties of these composites with the proportion of carbon fibers in the composites, it is possible to modify the material design flexibility to suit the ultimate design of prostheses.

Composites have unique properties and are usually stronger than any of the single materials from which they are made. Workers in this field have taken advantages of this fact and applied it to some difficult problems where tissue in-growth is necessary. Examples:

> Deposited Al_2O_3 onto carbon;
>
> Carbon / PTFE;
>
> Al_2O_3 / PTFE;
>
> PLA- coated Carbon fibers.

Ceramics

The most frequently used ceramic implant materials include aluminum oxides, calcium phosphates, and apatites and graphite. Glasses have also been developed for medical applications. The use of ceramics was motivated by:

- their inertness in the body,
- their formability into a variety of shapes and porosities,
- their high compressive strength, and
- some cases their excellent wear characteristics.

Selected applications of ceramics include:

- hip prostheses,
- artificial knees,
- bone grafts,
- a variety of tissues in growth related applications in
    1. (d.1) orthopedics
    2. (d.2) dentistry, and
    3. (d.3) heart valves.

Applications of ceramics are in some cases limited by their generally poor mechanical properties: (a) in tension; (b) load bearing, implant devices that are to be subjected to significant tensile stresses must be designed and manufactured with great care if ceramics are to be safely used.

Biodegradable Materials

Another class of materials that is receiving increased attention is biodegradable materials. Generally, when a material degrades in the body its properties change from their original values leading to altered and less desirable performance. It is possible, however, to design into an implant's performance the controlled degradation of a material, such that natural tissue replaces the prosthesis and its function.

Examples include: Suture material that hold a wound together but resorb in the body as the wound heals and gains strength. Another application of these materials occurs when they are used to encourage natural tissue to grow. Certain wound dressings and ceramic bone augmentation materials encourage tissue to grow into them by providing a "scaffold". The scaffold material may or may not resorb over a period of time but in each case, natural tissue has grown into the space, then by restoring natural function. One final application of biodegradable materials is in drug therapy, where it is possible to chemically bond certain drugs to the biodegradable material, when these materials are placed within the body the drug is released as the material degrades, thereby providing a localized, sustained release of drugs over a predictable period of time.

Mechanical Properties of Biomaterials

The tensile test is a common testing procedure used to provide data for characterization of biomaterials. The discussion below focuses on special considerations needed for tensile testing biological soft tissue (e.g. ligament and tendon) compared to traditional engineering materials (e.g. aluminum and steel).

- Traditional Engineering Materials

  Common assumptions used for testing and analysis of traditional materials are that they are homogeneous, exhibit small deformations and are linearly elastic. Young's modulus (E), the slope of the elastic portion of stress-strain curve, is a quantity often used to assess a material stiffness. The linear elastic assumption makes the determination of "E" relatively straight-forward as it can be assessed anywhere along the initial linear portion of the curve.

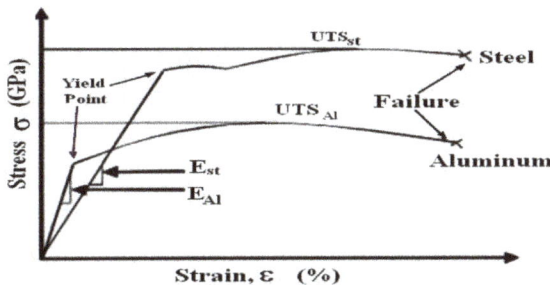

Figure: Stress-strain curve of traditional engineering materials

- Biological Soft Tissue Materials

  The assumptions made for the traditional materials are not valid when testing biological soft tissue samples. These materials are, in general, non- homogeneous due to the orientation of their collagen and elastin fibers. Hence, care must be taken when collecting samples and positioning them in testing system to ensure the directions are consistent with the intended analysis. Biological tissues exhibit large deformation before failure, therefore, any transducer used to measure strain will need to accommodate the large movement. Due to the un-crimping of collagen fibers and elasticity of elastin, the initial portion of a biological sample stress-strain curve has a high deformation/low force characteristics known as the toe region. In short, unlike traditional materials, this region is non-linear. A linear region is typically identified after the toe region and is used for the determination of E.

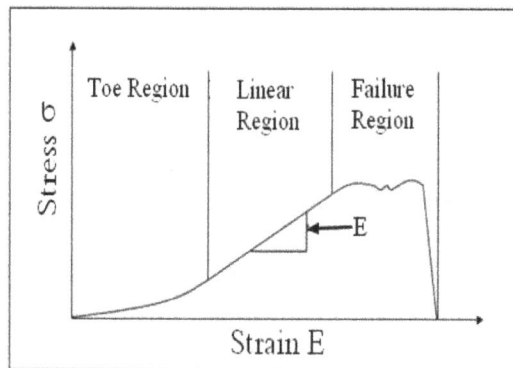

Figure: Stress-Strain Curve of Biological Soft Tissue Material

The mechanical properties of biological tissues are strain or loading rate dependent due to these tissues, visco-elastic nature. For example, biological tissues typically become stiffer with increasing strain rate.

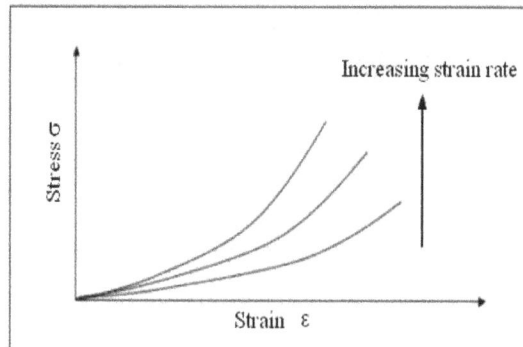

Figure: Strain rate Dependence

As such, predetermined and tightly controlled strain or loading rates must be maintained during testing. Furthermore, many biological tissues in their normal state are preconditioned (e.g. the anterior cruciate ligament) while many are not (e.g. brain).

For a tissue that has not been preconditioned, its response to load or displacement from one cycle to the next will not be similar; hence results will not be consisten.

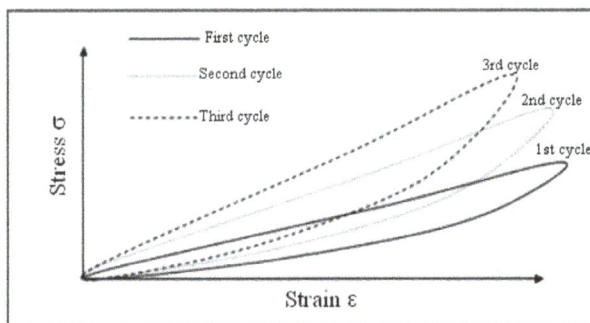

Figure: Preconditioning

Depending on the type of tissue being tested or response of interest (e.g. sudden impact or fatigue failure), preconditioning as part of the testing protocol may or may not be necessary.

Thermal Properties

Wide temperature fluctuations occur in the oral cavity due to the ingestion of hot or cold food and drink. Thermal Conductivity is the rate of heat flow per unit temperature gradient. Thus, good conductors have high values of conductivity.

Material	Thermal Conductivity
Enamel	$0.92 \ W.m^{-1}.^{0}C^{-1}$
Dentine	$\cdot.63 \ W.m^{-1}.^{0}C^{-1}$
Acrylic Resin	$0.21 \ W.m^{-1}.^{0}C^{-1}$
Dental Amalgam	$23.02 \ W.m^{-1}.^{0}C^{-1}$
Zinc Phosphate Cement	$1.17 \ W.m^{-1}.^{0}C^{-1}$
Zinc Oxide Cement	$0.46 \ W.m^{-1}.^{0}C^{-1}$
Silicate Materials	$0.75 \ W.m^{-1}.^{0}C^{-1}$
Porcelain	$1.05 \ W.m^{-1}.^{0}C^{-1}$
Gold	$291.70 \ W.m^{-1}.^{0}C^{-1}$

Thermal Diffusivity (D) is defined by the equation: $D = \dfrac{K}{C_p \rho}$

Where, K is thermal conductivity;

C_p is heat capacity, and

ρ is density.

Measurements of thermal diffusivity are often made by embedding a thermocouple in a specimen of material and plunging the specimen into hot or cold liquid. If the temperature, recorded by the thermocouple, rapidly reaches that of the liquid, this indicates a high value of diffusivity. A slow response indicates a lower value of diffusivity is preferred. In many circumstances, a low value of diffusivity is preferred. There are occasions on which a high value is beneficial. For example, a denture base material, ideally, should have a high value of thermal diffusivity in order that the patient retains a satisfactory response to hot and cold stimuli in the mouth.

Coefficient of Thermal Expansion is defined as the fractional increase in length of a body for each degree centigrade increase in temperature.

$$\alpha = \frac{\Delta L / L_0}{\Delta T} \ {}^0C^{-1}$$

Where ΔL is the change in length;

L_0 is the original length;

ΔT is the temperature change.

Because the values of α very small numbers. For example for amalgam

$\alpha = 0.0000025 \ {}^{\circ}C^{-1} = 25 \ {}^{\circ}C^{-1}$ p.p.m (partpermillion).

Material	Coefficient of thermal expansion (p.p.m. ${}^0C^{-1}$)
Enamel	11.4
Dentine	8.0
Acrylic Resin	90.0
Porcelain	4.0
Amalgam	25.0
Composite resins	25 – 60
Silicate Cements	10.0

This property is particularly important for filling materials. For filling materials, the most ideal combination of properties would be low value of diffusivity combined with (a) similar to that for tooth substance.

Chemical Properties

One of the main factors, which determine the durability of a material, is its chemical stability. Material should not dissolve, erode or corrode, nor should they leach important constituents into oral fluids.

- Solubility and Erosion

The solubility of a material is a measurement of the extent to which it will dissolve in a given fluid, for example, water or saliva. Erosion is a process which combines the chemical process of dissolution with a mild mechanical action.

These properties are particularly important for all restorative materials since a high solubility or poor resistance to erosion will severely limit the effective lifetime of the restoration.

The pH of oral fluids may vary from pH4 to pH8.5, representing a range from mildly acidic to mildly alkaline. Highly acidic soft drinks and the use of chalk-containing tooth-pastes extend this range from a lower end of pH2 up to pH11. It is possible for a material to be stable at near neutral pH7 values but to erode rapidly at extremes of either acidity or alkalinity.

Standard tests of solubility often involve the storage of disc specimens of materials in water for a period of time, the results being quoted as the percentage weight loss of the disc. Such methods, however, often give misleading results.

When comparing silicate and phosphate cements, for example, silicate materials appear more soluble in simple laboratory test, but in practice they are more durable than the phosphates.

- Leaching of Constituents

Many materials, when placed in an aqueous environment, absorb water by a diffusion process. Constituents of the material may be lost into the oral fluids by a diffusion process commonly referred to as leaching.

Some soft acrylic polymers, used for cushioning, the fitting surfaces of dentures rely on the absence of relatively large quantities of plasticizer in the acrylic resin for their softness. The slow leaching of plasticizer causes the resin to become hard and, therefore, ineffective as a cushion.

Occasionally, leaching is used to the benefit of the patient. For example, in some cements containing calcium hydroxide, slow leaching causes an alkaline environment in the base of deep cavities. This has the dual benefit of being antibacterial and of encouraging secondary dentine formation.

- Corrosion

It is a term which specifically characterizes the chemical reactivity of metals and alloys. Metals and alloys are good electrical conductors and many corrosion processes involve the setting up of an electrolytic cell as a first stage in the process.

The tendency of a metal to corrode can be predicted from its electrode potential. It can be seen from the figure, that materials with large negative electrode potential values are more reactive whilst those with large positive values are far less reactive and are often referred to as noble metals.

```
                              Gold
                            Platinum
        +ve Electrode        Silver
           Potential         Mercury
                             Copper
                            Hydrogen      Increasing      Increasing
                              Iron         Nobility        Reactivity
                              Tin
        -ve Electrode       Chromium
           Potential          Zinc
                            Aluminum
                             Calcium
```

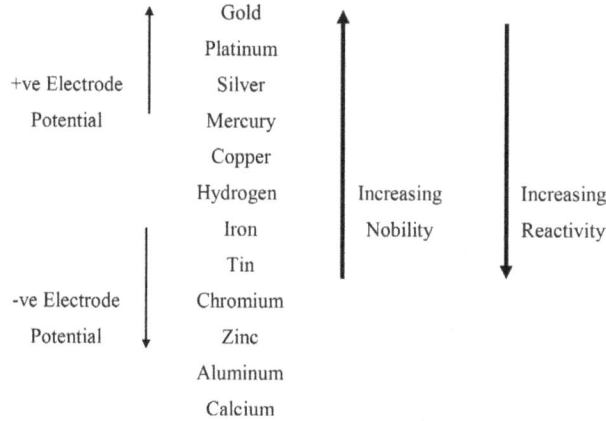

It can be seen that chromium has a negative value of electrolytic potential and is at the reactive end of the series of metals shown. It is, therefore, surprising to learn that chromium is included as a component of many alloys in order to improve corrosion resistance. The apparent contradiction can be explained by the passivating effect. Although chromium is electrochemically active it reacts readily forming a layer of chromic oxide, which protects the metal or alloy from further decomposition.

Other factors, which can affect the corrosion of metals and alloys, are stress and surface roughness. Stress in metal components of appliances produces, for example, by excessive or continued bending can accelerate the rate of corrosion and may lead to failure by stress corrosion cracking.

Pits in rough surfaces can lead to the setting up of small corrosion cells in which the material at the bottom of the pit acts as the anode and that at the surface acts as the cathode. The mechanism of this type of corrosion sometimes referred to as concentration cell corrosion, is complicated but is caused by the fact that pits tend to become filled with debris, which reduces the oxygen concentration in the base of the pit compared with the surface. In order to reduce corrosion by this new mechanism, metals and alloys used in the mouth should be polished to remove surface irregularities.

Ideally, a material placed into a patient's mouth should be non-toxic, nonirritant, have no carcinogenic or allergic potential and if used as a filling material, should be harmless to the pulp.

Doctors, researchers, and bioengineers use biomaterials for the following broad range of applications:

- Medical implants, including heart valves, stents, and grafts; artificial joints, ligaments, and tendons; hearing loss implants; dental implants; and devices that stimulate nerves.

- Methods to promote healing of human tissues, including sutures, clips, and staples for wound closure, and dissolvable dressings.

- Regenerated human tissues, using a combination of biomaterial supports or scaffolds, cells, and bioactive molecules. Examples include a bone regenerating hydrogel and a lab-grown human bladder.

- Molecular probes and nanoparticles that break through biological barriers and aid in cancer imaging and therapy at the molecular level.

- Biosensors to detect the presence and amount of specific substances and to transmit that data. Examples are blood glucose monitoring devices and brain activity sensors.

- Drug-delivery systems that carry and/or apply drugs to a disease target. Examples include drug-coated vascular stents and implantable chemotherapy wafers for cancer patients.

Biocompatibility

Biocompatibility is determined as the ability of a material to co-exist and perform with a natural substance in a specific biological application. Since the material should be non-toxic to perform with an appropriate host response, which having a biomaterial interface with human body are required to perform a particular physiological function such as that of stent, knee replacement or pacemaker. Biomaterials incorporated into medical devices are implanted into tissues and organs. Therefore, the key principles governing the structure of normal and abnormal cells, tissues and organs, the techniques by which the structure and function of normal and abnormal tissue are studied, and the fundamental mechanisms of disease processes are critical considerations. Special processes are invoked when a material or device heals in the body. Injury to tissue will stimulate the well-defined inflammatory reaction sequence that leads to healing. Where a foreign body (e.g., an implant) is present in the wound site (surgical incision), the reaction sequence is referred to as the "foreign body reaction." The normal response of the body will be modulated because of the solid implant. Furthermore, this reaction will differ in intensity and duration depending upon the anatomical site involved. An understanding of how a foreign object alters the normal inflammatory reaction sequence remain an important concern.

It is a measurement of how compatible a device is with a biological system. The purpose of performing biocompatibility testing is to determine the fitness of a device for human use, and to see whether use of the device can have any potentially harmful physiological effects.

Typically, material characterization and analysis of a device's components are conducted prior to any biological testing. This involves extracting leachable materials from the device or components at an elevated temperature, and analyzing the leachable extracts for potentially harmful chemicals or cytotoxicity.

Once in vitro testing has been completed, in vivo biological testing can be done based upon the device's intended use. This testing can range from skin irritation testing to hemocompatibility and implantation testing. Turnaround time for tests can range from three weeks to greater than several months, depending on the specific test data needed. Subchronic or chronic implantation testing can last even longer. The two ways to test the biocompatibility in vivo implant are "Tissue culture test" and "Blood and contact tests".

Table: Examples of Biomaterials application in medical devices

1	Joint replacements
2	Bone plates
3	Bone cement
4	Artificial ligaments and tendons
5	Dental implants for tooth fixation
6	Blood vessel prostheses
7	Heart valves
8	Skin repair devices (artificial tissue)
9	Cochlear replacement
10	Contact lenses
11	Breast implants
12	Drug delivery mechanisms
13	Sustainable materials
14	Vascular grafts
15	Stents
16	Nerve Conduits

Some commonly used Biomaterials are given below:

Material categorizes	Applications
Silicone rubber	Catheters, tubing
Dacron	Vascular grafts
Cellulose	Dialysis membranes
Poly (methyl methacrylate)	Intraocular lenses, bone cement
Polyurethanes	Catheters, pacemaker leads
Hydogels	Ophthalmological devices, Drug Delivery
Stainless steel	orthopedic devices, stents
Titanium	Orthopedic and dental devices
Alumina	Orthopedic and dental devices
Hydroxyapatite	Orthopedic and dental devices
Collagen (reprocessed)	Opthalmologic applications, wound dressings

A biomaterial should not be toxic, unless it is specifically engineered for such requirements (for example, a "smart bomb" drug delivery system that targets cancer cells and destroys them). Since the nontoxic requirement is the norm, toxicology for biomaterials has evolved into a sophisticated science. It deals with the substances that migrate out of biomaterials. For example, for polymers, many low-molecular-weight "leachables" exhibit some level of physiologic activity and cell toxicity. It is reasonable to say that a biomaterial should not give off anything from its mass unless it is specifically designed to do so. Toxicology also deals with methods to evaluate how well this design criterion is met when a new biomaterial is under development.

Mechanical and Performance Requirements

An intraocular lens may go into the lens capsule or the anterior chamber of the eye. A hip joint will be implanted in bone across an articulating joint space. A heart valve will be sutured into cardiac muscle and will contact both soft tissue and blood. A catheter may be placed in an artery, a vein or the urinary tract. Each of these sites challenges the biomedical device designer with special requirements for geometry, size, mechanical properties, and bioresponses.

Biomaterials and devices have mechanical and performance requirements that originate from the physical and /or electrochemical properties of the material. Such requirement varies in mechanical properties for example:

Hip prosthesis must be strong and rigid, tendon material must be strong and flexible, heart valve leaflet must be flexible and tough, dialysis membrane must be strong and flexible, but not elastomeric, articular cartilage substitute must be soft and elastomeric.

Then, mechanical performance varies based on a diverse range of requirements. Similarly the duration of contact also varies, for example :-

A catheter may be required for just 3 days, bone plate may fulfill its function in 6 months or longer, leaflet in a heart valve must flex 60 times per minute without tearing for the lifetime of the patient (realistically, at least for 10 or more years), hip joint must not fail under heavy loads for more than 10 years and so on. There are also other biophysical properties and other aspects of performance. The dialysis membrane has a specified permeability, the articular cup of the hip joint must have high lubricity, and the intraocular lens has clarity and refraction requirements. To meet these requirements, design principles from physics, chemistry, mechanical engineering, chemical engineering, and materials science are to be accurately integrated.

Regulation

Patient care demands safe medical devices. To prevent inadequately tested devices and materials from coming on the market. Most nations of the world have medical device regulatory bodies. In addition the International Standards Organization (ISO) has introduced international standards for the world community. The costs to comply with the standards and to implement materials, biological, and clinical testing are enormous. As per regulatory requirement testing and other factors involved in biomaterials can be categorized as below:

Table: Requirements of Implants

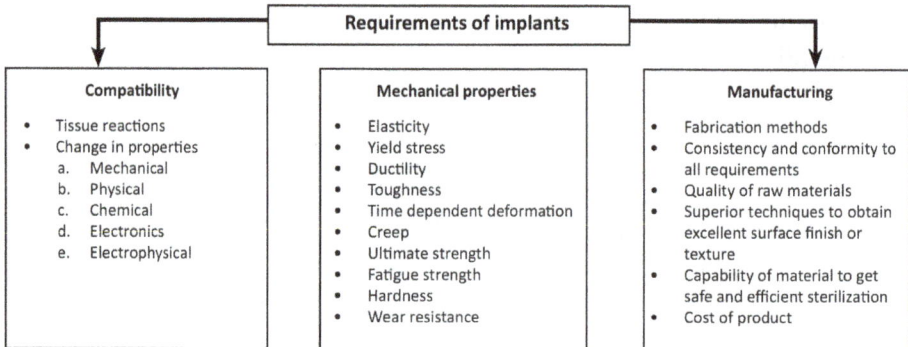

Requirements of implants		
Compatibility	**Mechanical properties**	**Manufacturing**

• Tissue reactions
• Change in properties
  a. Mechanical
  b. Physical
  c. Chemical
  d. Electronics
  e. Electrophysical
	• Elasticity
	• Yield stress
	• Ductility
	• Toughness
	• Time dependent deformation
	• Creep
	• Ultimate strength
	• Fatigue strength
	• Hardness
	• Wear resistance
		• Fabrication methods
		• Consistency and conformity to all requirements
		• Quality of raw materials
		• Superior techniques to obtain excellent surface finish or texture
		• Capability of material to get safe and efficient sterilization
		• Cost of product

Nanocellulose

Nanocellulose is a light solid substance obtained from plant matter which comprises nanosized cellulose fibrils. This new material is a pseudo-plastic and possesses the property of specific kinds of fluids or gels that are generally thick in normal conditions. The lateral dimensions of nanocellulose range from 5 to 20 nm, and the longitudinal dimension ranges from a few 10's of nanometers to several microns.

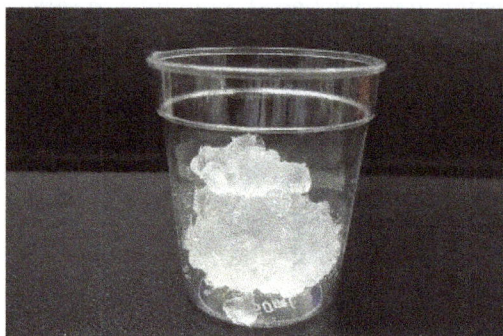

Figure: *Nanocellulose is transparent, electrically conductive, and stronger than steel.*

Properties of Nanocellulose

The properties of nanocellulose are listed below:

- Lightweight
- Stiffer than Kevlar

- Electrically conductive

- Non-toxic

- The crystalline form is transparent, and gas impermeable

- It can be produced in large quantities in a cost-effective manner

- It has a very high tensile strength - 8 times that of steel

- It is highly absorbent when used as a basis for aerogels or foams.

- The raw material - cellulose - is the most abundant polymer on earth

Type of Nanocellulose

Cellulose Nanocrystals

Cellulose nanocrystals (CNCs) are commonly produced using acid hydrolysis of cellulosic materials dispersed in water. In general, concentrated sulfuric acid is used, which dissolves the amorphous regions of cellulose and the crystalline regions are left alone. Although this technique produces a rod-like rigid CNC with almost 90% purity, the sulfate groups remain attached at the surface of the fibers as impurities. The length and diameter of CNCs commonly vary from a length of 200–500 nm to a diameter of 3–35 nm.

Cellulose Nanofibrils

CNFs are long entangled fibrils (μm) with a diameter in nanometer range. CNFs are produced by high-pressure grinding of cellulosic pulp suspension and strongly entangled networks of nanofibrils are formed . Unlike CNCs, which have near-perfect crystallinity, CNFs contain both amorphous as well as crystalline cellulose domains within the single fibers. Typically, CNFs have a diameter of 5–50 nm and a length of a few micrometers. CNF extraction from cellulosic fibers can be obtained by three types of processes: (1) mechanical treatments (e.g., homogenization, grinding, and milling); (2) chemical treatments (e.g., TEMPO oxidation); and (3) a combination of chemical and mechanical treatments.

Bacterial Cellulose

Bacterial cellulose (BC) is also known as microbial cellulose. It is typically produced from bacteria, (e.g., Acetobacterxylinum) as a separate molecule and does not require additional processing to remove contaminants like lignin, pectin, and hemicellulose. Furthermore in contrast to CNC and CNF biosynthesis, BC biosynthesis involves the addition of molecules from tiny units (Å) to small units (nm). In the biosynthesis of BC, the glucose chains are supplied inside the bacterial body and expelled out through minor pores present on the cell wall. Ribbon-shaped BC nanofibers are formed when glucose is combined with the cell wall. This ribbon-like web-shaped structure produces a 20–100 nm long unique nanofiber system.

Preparation Methods/Nanocellulose Synthesis Methods

Pretreatment Methods

Pretreatment of wood cellulose fibers is a technique to reduce the energy consumption of mechanical nanofibrillation processes to improve the degree of nanofibrillation. Since energy consumption is the main drawback for the production of nanofibers by mechanical isolation processes, the pretreatment process has become an important step. Furthermore it improves the fibrillation process with increase in production of nanofibers.

Enzyme Hydrolysis

Enzymes with the ability of selective hydrolysis, such as laccase, can degrade or modify the lignin and hemicellulose contents without disturbing cellulose content. Since cellulosic fibers contain many different organic compounds as a composite structure, a single specific enzyme cannot degrade the fiber. The following sets of enzymes are required to decay extra cellulose compound:

1. Cellobiohydrolases: A & B type cellulases—attack greatly on crystalline cellulose

2. Endoglucanases: C & D type cellulases—attack disordered structure of cellulose

Pääkkö and Ankerfors produced NFC from bleached softwood pulp. In this method a mild enzymatic hydrolysis was applied followed by refining and homogenization. It was observed that the mild hydrolysis using endoglucanase increased the aspect ratio without a harsh reaction compared to acid hydrolysis. An additional advantage of enzyme pretreatment is that it increases the solids level, which allows a smooth pass during HPH processing. Furthermore they showed a higher aspect ratio and more distinct compared to untreated.

Alkaline–Acid

Alkaline–acid pretreatment is the most common method used for lignin, hemicellulose, and pectin solubilization before mechanical isolation of NFC. This method included the following steps:

1. Sodium hydroxides (NaOH)- Soaking fibers in 12–17.5 wt% solution for 2 hours. This raises the surface area of cellulosic fibers and eases the hydrolysis.

2. Hydrochloric acid (HCL)- Soaking fibers in 1 M solution at 60–80°C. This solubilizes the hemicelluloses.

3. Sodium hydroxides (NaOH)- Treating with 2 wt% solution for 2 hours at 60–80°C. This disrupts the lignin structure, and breaks the linkages between carbohydrate and lignin. Alkaline pretreatment is an effective method that can improve cellulose yield from 43% to 84%. It also helps to removed lignin and hemicelluloses partially from soy hull fibers and wheat straw.

Ionic Liquids

Ionic liquids (ILs) are organic salts having special properties such as nonflammability, thermal and chemical stability, and infinitely low vapor pressure. It is an increasing interest of researchers to study as solvents of cellulosic materials. Li, Wei treated sugarcane bagasse with 1-butyl-3-methylimidazolium chloride [(Bmim) Cl] as ionic liquid and followed the high-pressure homogenization (HPH) technique to prepare NFC. The pulp passed through homogenizer without clogging; these fibers were then precipitated in water solution and regenerated by freeze-drying.

Mechanical Process

Cellulosic materials are required to go through mechanical treatment for defibrillation. Pretreatment processing, either by chemicals or enzymes, is done before mechanical fibrillation to ease the process. Chemical treatments help in widening the space between hydroxyl groups, increasing the inner surface, altering crystallinity, and breaking cellulose hydrogen bonds, thus enhancing surface areas, which help boost the reactivity of the fibers. There are many mechanical methods for converting cellulosic fiber to nanocellulose, such as homogenizing, microfluidization, grinding, cryocrushing, and high-intensity ultrasonication (HIUS).

High-pressure Homogenization

High-pressure homogenization (HPH) is an efficient method for refining of cellulosic fibers. It was introduced in 1983, to use nanofibril cellulose from wood pulp. This procedure is very simple and does not involve addition of any organic solvents. In this process, cellulosic pulp is passed through a very small nozzle at high pressure. There are many types of forces that can be applied on cellulose pulp such as high velocity and pressure, as well as impact and shear forces, which influence fluid to generate shear rates in the stream and decrease the size of fibers to the nanoscale. Many researchers have used HPH for many other raw materials, such as bleached sugar beet extraction of prickly pear, etc. There are some drawbacks in HPH, such as fiber clogging. Cellulosic fibers must be chopped very small and passed through HPH to avoid this problem. Mechanical pre-treatments are before HPH to produce nanofibers from kenaf bast fiber.

Microfluidization

Microfluidizers work similar to HPH in the production of nanocellulose fiber. Microfluidizers use an intensifier pump to enhance pressure, while the interaction chamber is used for shear and impact forces against colliding streams to defibril- late the fibers. The cellulose fibrils showed a higher amount of hydroxyl (OH) groups as well as agglomeration behavior due to more surface area. The number of passes through the homogenizer determines the size of NFC and its surface area.

Grinding

Grinding is another strategy to break up cellulose into nanosize fibers. In this process, pulp passes through a couple of stones, where one stone is fixed while the other stone rotates. This mechanism provides shear forces to break down the hydrogen bond and cell wall structure of fibers and convert pulp into nanoscale fibers. Wang and Drzal used a commercial stone grinder to produce NFC from bleached eucalyptus pulp, which helps to study the relation between energy consumption and fibrillation time as a function of crystallinity. Friction of stones generates heat due to the fibrillation process, which helps to evaporate water content and raise solid content, which takes 11 hours to boost specific fibrillation energy. Number of cycles through HPH and grinding processes affects the characterization of resultant NFC. In HPH, pulp fiber is passed through 30 times but 14 repetitions showed effective results; in the case of grinding, 10 cycles are recommended to create uniform size of NFC.

Cryocrushing

Cryocrushing is another mechanical method used to break the cellulose wall into nanosize fibers. In this method, fibers are kept in water and cellulose absorbs water in its cavity. Water-soaked cellulose is immersed in liquid nitrogen, which solidifies the water content, and is subsequently crushed by mortar and pestle. Applying high-impact force on frozen cellulosic fibers leads to rupture due to applied pressure through ice crystals resulting in conversion to nanocellulose. Wang and Sain studied the HPH and cryocrushing processes to produce nanofibers from soybean stock and observed the diameter of nanofibers in the range of 50–100 nm through transmission electron microscopy (TEM).

High-intensity Ultrasonication

The HIUS process uses hydrodynamic forces of ultrasound with oscillation power to isolate cellulose fibrils. In this process, cavities in cells of cellulose convert into powerful mechanical oscillating power. Molecules absorb the ultrasonic energy of high-intensity waves and consist of formation, expansion, and implosion of microscopic gas bubbles. Various studies have been reported dealing with the synthesis of nanocellulose fiber from cellulose through HIUS and oscillating power. It was concluded that high temperature, high power, and short fiber size are required to make better fibrillation. It is also reported that a combination of HPH and HIUS increased the fibrillation and provided uniformity in nanofibers compared to HIUS alone.

Ball Milling Process

Ball milling is a mechanical process in which cellulose suspension is placed in a hollow cylindrical container for the production of CNF. This hollow cylindrical container is partially filled with balls made up of ceramic, zirconia, or metal; the container rotates and breaks cellulose cell walls through the high-energy collision between the balls. Maintaining homogeneity of the produced CNF is always a major challenge in this method.

Chemical Hydrolysis

The NFCs produced by mechanical methods consist of alternating crystalline and amorphous regions within the single cellulose domains. In order to dissolve the amorphous domain and permit longitudinal cutting of microfibrils, strong but controlled acid hydrolysis treatment is performed. The obtained nanocellulose, as aqueous suspension exhibits crystallinity greater than 90%, is termed as CNCs. In the acid hydrolysis process, the hydronium ion enters the amorphous regions of cellulose chains and promotes the hydrolytic cleavage of the glycosidic bonds. A mechanical treatment for nanocellulose dispersion, such as sonication, is required to prevent agglomeration. Various strong acids have been studied successfully to degrade cellulose fiber but the most common are hydrochloric and sulfuric acids. However, for the preparation of crystalline cellulosic nanoparticles, phosphoric acid , as well as hydrobromic and nitric acids , were recommended. The benefit of using sulfuric acid as hydrolyzing agent is it initiates the esterification process on the cellulose surface and promotes the grafting of anionic sulfate ester groups. Furthermore, the presence of anion groups induces the formation of a negative electrostatic layer on the surface of the nanocrystals and helps their dispersion in water. However, it reduces the agglomeration and reduces the thermostability of the nanoparticles . The reduced thermal stability of H_2SO_4-prepared CNCs can be improved by neutralizing by sodium hydroxide. Although these nanoparticles possess high-aspect-ratio, rod-like nanocrystals, their geometrical dimensions depend on the source of cellulose and hydrolysis methods. The length of the CNCs varies widely in the range of a few hundred nanometers due to the diffusion control nature of the acid hydrolysis, while the width is in the range of nanometers. Acid hydrolysis is the easiest and oldest method of CNC preparation.

Application

Nanocellulose is believed to be replacements for synthetic materials in more environ-mentally friendly materials, and is an addition to completely new types of biomaterials, i.e., cellulose nanocomposites. Nowadays, cellulose nanocomposites are being used in medical, automotive, electronics, packaging, construction, and wastewater treatment applications.

Nanocellulose in the Paper Industry

The papermaking process involves steps including preparing the paper components, wet refining, forming of wet sheet, pressing, drying, calendering, and finishing. Refining of cellulose fibers in water medium is a mandatory step in papermaking in order to obtain strong paper. Recent developments by Ioelvich and Leykin have shown the likelihood to increase the strength of paper with additive of nanocellulose particles to paper compositions. Such sheets exhibit admirable mechanical properties.

Nanocellulose in the Composite Industry

In recent years, there has been a remarkable growth in interest in the use of nanocellulose as polymer reinforcement in order to create high-performance biomaterials. The core reason for the appeal of nanosized cellulose is that material with higher uniformity and fewer defects with enhanced mechanical properties can be achieved by reducing the size of the cellulose fiber. It can be used as a reinforcing filler to prepare composites with solutions of water-soluble polymers to modify the viscosity and increase mechanical properties of dry composites. Of utmost importance has been the addition of nanocellulose to biodegradable polymers, which permits both the improvement of mechanical properties and speeds up the rate of biodegradation.

Nanocellulose in the Biomedical Industry

Nanocellulose is a natural biodegradable material, highly suitable for the biomedical industry. Pure nanocellulose is nontoxic for people and it is biocompatible. For that reason, it can be utilized for health care applications such as personal hygiene products, cosmetics, and biomedicines. One of the most modest applications of nano-cellulose is in the stabilization of medical suspensions against phase separation and sedimentation of heavy ingredients. Chemically modified cellulose can be a promising carrier for immobilization of enzymes and other drugs. Due to its nanosize, such a carrier-drug complex can penetrate through skin pores and treat skin diseases. Likewise, it can be used as a gentle but active peeling agent in cosmetics.

Bioceramic

Ceramic is defined as "synthesized inorganic, solid, crystalline materials, excluding metals". Ceramics, used as biomaterials to fill defects in tooth and bone, to fix bone grafts, fractures, or prostheses to bone, and to replace diseased tissue, are called bioceramics. They must be highly biocompatible and anti thrombogenic, and should not be toxic, allergenic, carcinogenic, or teratogenic. Bioceramics can be classified into three groups; (1) bioinert ceramics, (2) bioactive ceramics, and (3) bioresorbable ceramics. Bioinert ceramics have a high chemical stability in vivo as well as high mechanical strength as a rule, and when they are implanted in living bone, they are incorporated into the bone tissue in accordance with the pattern of "contact osteogenesis". On the other hand, bioactive ceramics have the character of osteoconduction and the capability of chemical bonding with living bone tissue. In other words, when bioactive ceramics are implanted in living bone, they are incorporated into the bone tissue in accordance with the pattern of "bonding osteogenesis". The mechanical strength of bioactive ceramics is generally lower than that of bioinert ceramics. Bioresorbable ceramics are gradually absorbed in vivo and replaced by bone in the bone tissue. The pattern of their incorporation into the bone tissue is considered similar to contact osteogenesis, although the interface between bioresorbable ceramics and bone is not stable as that observed with bioinert ceramics.

Bioinert Ceramics

Ceramics are fully oxidized materials and are therefore chemically very stable. Thus ceramics are less likely to elicit an adverse biological response than metals, which only oxidize at their surface. Three types of inert ceramics are of interest in musculoskeletal applications: carbon, alumina, and zirconia.

Carbon

The benign biological reaction elicited by carbon-based materials, along with the similarity in stiff- ness and strength between carbon and bone, made carbon a candidate material for musculoskeletal reconstruction. Carbon has a hexagonal crystal structure that is formed by strong covalent bonds. Graphite has a planar hexagonal array structure with a crystal size of approximately 1000 Å. The carbon-carbon bond energy within the planes is large, whereas the bond between the planes is weak. Therefore, carbon derives its strength from the strong in-plane bonds, whereas the weak bonding between the planes results in a low modulus, near that of bone.

Isotropic carbon, on the other hand, has no preferred crystal orientation and hence possesses isotropic material properties. There are three types of isotropic carbon: pyrolytic, vitreous, and vapor- deposited carbon. Pyrolytic carbons are formed by the deposition of carbon from a fluidized bed onto a substrate. The fluidized bed is formed from pyrolysis of hydrocarbon gas at between 1000 and 2500°C. Low-temperature isotropic (LTI) carbons are formed at temperatures below 1500°C. LTI pyrolytic carbon possesses good frictional and wear properties, and incorporation of silicon can further increase hardness and wear resistance.

Vitreous carbon is a fine-grained polycrystalline material formed by slow heating of a polymer. On heating, the more volatile components diffuse from the structure, and only carbon remains. Since the process is diffusion-mediated and potentially volatile, heating must be slow, and the dimensions of the structure are therefore limited to approximately 7 mm.

Attempts have been made at depositing LTI coatings onto metallic substrates. The limiting factor in these systems was the brittleness of the carbon coating and the propensity for coating fracture and coating-substrate debonding. Carbon may also be vapor deposited onto a substrate by the evaporation of carbon atoms from a high-temperature source and subsequent condensation onto a low-temperature substrate. Vapor-deposited coatings are typically about 1 μm thick. As a result, the bulk properties of the substrate are retained. More recently, diamondlike carbon (DLC) coatings have been studied, primarily as a means of improving wear and corrosion resistance of articulating components of joint replacement. Carbon-based thin films are produced from solid carbon or liquid/gaseous hydrocarbon sources using ion-beam or plasma-deposition techniques. Resulting coatings are metastable amorphous with properties intermediate to those of graphite and diamond.

Alumina

High-density, high-purity polycrystalline alumina is used for femoral stems, femoral heads, acetabular components, and dental implants. More recently, ion-modified and nanostructured forms of Al_2O_3 have been synthesized in attempts to make these traditionally inert bioceramics more bioactive. The attributes of alumina, aside from its chemical stability and relative biologic inertness, are its hardness and excellent friction and wear resistance. As a result, a main motivation for using alumina in reconstructive surgery has been for tribologic improvements, and many total hip replace- ments are now designed as modular devices; i.e., an alumina femoral head is press-fit onto the neck of a metallic femoral stem. The alumina head then articulates in either a polyethylene or alumina acetabular cup.

Table: Physical and Mechanical Properties of Bioceramics

Material	Porosity, %	Density, mg/m³	Modulus, GPa	Compressive strength MPa	Tensile strength MPa	Flexural strength MPa	K_{Ic}, MPa·m$^{1/2}$
Graphite	7	1.8	25	—	—	140	—
(isotropic)	12	1.8	20–24	65–95	24–30	45–55	—
	16–20	1.6–1.85	6–13.4	18–58	8–19	14–27	—
	30	1.55	7.1	—	—	—	—
	—	0.1–0.5	—	2.5–30	—	—	—
Pyrolytic	2.7	2.19	28–41	—	—	—	—
graphite, LTI	—	1.3–2	17–28	900	200	340–520	—
	—	1.7–2.2	17–28	—	—	270–550	—
Glassy (vitreous)	—	1.4–1.6	—	—	—	70–205	—
carbon	—	1.45–1.5	24–28	700	70–200	150–200	—
	—	1.38–1.4	23–29	—	—	190–255	—
	≤50	<1.1	7–32	50–330	13–52	—	—
Bioactive	—	—	—	—	56–83	—	—
ceramics and	—	2.8	—	500	—	100–150	—
glass ceramics	31–76	0.65–1.86	2.2–21.8	—	—	4–35	—
Hydroxyapatite	0.1–3	3.05–3.15	7–13	350–450	38–48	100–120	—
	10	2.7	—	—	—	—	—
	30	—	—	120–170	—	—	—
	40	—	—	60–120	—	15–35	—
	2.8–19.4	2.55–3.07	44–48	310–510	—	60–115	—
	2.5–26.5	—	55–110	≤800	—	50–115	—
Tetracalcium-phosphate	Dense	3.1	—	120–200	—	—	—
Tricalcium-phosphate	Dense	3.14	—	120	—	—	—
Other calcium phosphates	Dense	2.8–3.1	—	70–170	—	—	—
Al_2O_3	0	3.93–3.95	380–400	4000–5000	350	400–500	5–6
	25	2.8–3.0	150	500	—	70	—
	35	—	—	200	—	55	—
	50–75	—	—	80	—	6–11.4	—
ZrO_2, stabilized	0	4.9–5.6	150–200	1750	—	150–900	4–12
(~ 3% Y_2O_3)	1.5	5.75	210–240	—	—	280–450	—
	5	—	150–200	—	—	50–500	—
	28	3.9–4.1	—	<400	—	50–65	—

High-purity alumina powder, prepared by calcining alumina trihydrate, is typically iso-statically compacted and shaped. Subsequent sintering at temperatures in the range 1600 to 1800°C transforms a preform into a dense polycrystalline solid having a grain size of less than 5 μm. Addition of trace amounts of MgO aids in sintering and limits grain growth. If processing is kept below 2050°C, a-Al_2O_3, which is the most stable phase, forms. Alternatively, single crystals (sapphire) may be grown by feeding powder onto a seed and allowing buildup.

The physical and mechanical properties (i.e., ultimate strength, fatigue strength, frac-ture toughness, and wear resistance) of a-alumina are a function of purity, grain size, grain size distribution, porosity, and inclusions. Both grain size d and porosity P (o = P = 1) affect strength s via well-characterized relations, where so is the strength of the dense ceramic and A, n and B are material constants, experimentally determined, with n typically approximately0.5.

$$\sigma = Ad^{-n}$$

$$\sigma_p = \sigma_0 e^{-BP}$$

For example, decreasing grain size from 4 to 7 μm increases strength by approximate-ly 20 percent. Advanced ceramics processing now makes it possible to fabricate alu-mina with grain sizes on the order of 1 μm and a small grain size distribution, material characteristics that result in increased strength. The elastic modulus of fully dense alumina is two- to fourfold greater than that of metals commonly used in bone and joint reconstruction.

Sintering and annealing cycles and the subsequent cooling can lead to residual stresses in alumina. Microcrack nucleation occurs at locally high residual stresses and at pores, inclusions, segregated grain boundaries, and grain-boundary triple points. Further-more, if there is a wide distribution of grain sizes, the material anisotropy leads to a larger range of thermal expansions and higher residual stresses. The long-term me-chanical properties of ceramics, however, may be predicted through the use of fracture mechanics and statistical methods.

Environment also affects the mechanical properties of alumina. For example, fatigue strength is reduced in an aqueous environment due to subcritical crack growth, which is enhanced by water adsorption through hydrogen bonding of water molecules with oxygen in the Al_2O_3 lattice. The threshold stress for subcritical crack growth is also a function of processing and purity. For example, thermal cycling can lead to microcrack-ing, whereas CaO impurities compromise mechanical integrity.

The amount of wear in alumina-alumina couples can be as much as 10 times less than in a metal- polyethylene system depending on experimental conditions and surface roughness of the ceramic. The coefficient of friction of both alumina-alumina and alumina-polyethylene is less than that of metal-polyethylene because of alumina's low surface roughness and wettability.

The major limitation of alumina is that it possesses relatively low tensile and bending strengths and fracture toughness and, as a consequence, is sensitive to stress concentrations and overloading. Clinically retrieved alumina total hip replacements exhibit damage thought to be caused by fatigue, impact, or overload. Elevated contact and shear stresses, which lead to subsurface damage accumulation at microstructural defects and grain boundaries, have been implicated in the failure process. In general, a large number of ceramic failures can be attributed to materials processing or design deficiencies and can be minimized through better materials choice and quality control.

Based on clinical experience and retrieval analyses, implant geometries should have a sphericity of less than 1 μm and a radius tolerance between components of 7 to 10 μm. These specifications are based on the rationale that too small a gap between the components does not provide sufficient room for necessary lubrication or an escape route for alumina particles, whereas too large a gap increases contact pressures. To design around the low mechanical properties, a 32-mm femoral head and an acetabular cup with a minimum 44-mm outside diameter are recommended.

Zirconia

Yttrium oxide partially stabilized zirconia (YPSZ) has been advocated as an alternative to alumina. This class of ceramic has a higher toughness than alumina since it can be transformation toughened and is used in bulk form or as a coating. There are currently approximately 150,000 zirconia components in clinical use.

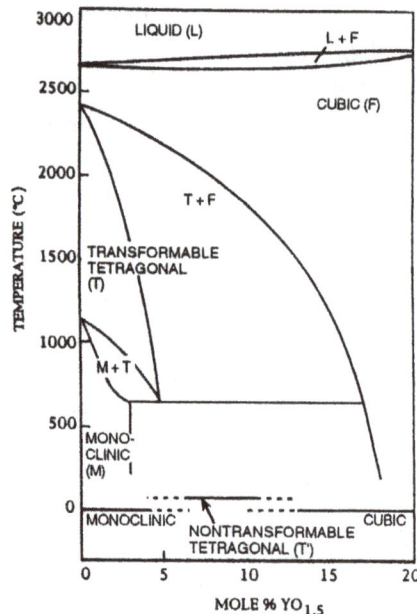

Figure: Schematic phase diagram of the $ZrO_2 - Y_2O_3$ system.

At room temperature, pure zirconia has monoclinic crystal symmetry and a density of 5.5 g/cm³. On heating, it transforms to a tetragonal phase (density ~ 6.1 g/cm³) at approximately 1000 to 1100°C and then to a cubic phase at approximately 2000°C. A partially reversible volumetric shrinkage (density increase) of 3 to 10 percent occurs during the monoclinic-to-tetragonal transformation. The volumetric changes resulting from the phase transformations can lead to residual stresses and cracking. Furthermore, because of the large volume reduction, pure zirconia cannot be sintered. However, sintering and phase transformations can be controlled via the addition of stabilizing oxides. Yttrium oxide (Y_2O_3) serves as a stabilizer for the tetragonal phase such that on cooling the tetragonal crystals are maintained in a metastable state and do not transform back to a monoclinic structure. The normal tetragonal-to-monoclinic transformation and volume change is additionally prevented by neighboring grains inducing compressive stresses on one another.

The modulus of partially stabilized zirconia is approximately half that of alumina, whereas the bending strength and fracture toughness are two to three and two times greater, respectively. The relatively high strength and toughness are a result of transformation toughening, a mechanism that manifests itself as follows: crack nucleation and propagation lead to locally elevated stresses and energy in the tetragonal crystals surrounding the crack tip. The elevated energy induces the metastable tetragonal grains to transform into monoclinic grains in this part of the microstructure. Since the monoclinic grains are larger than the tetragonal grains, there is a local volume increase, compressive stresses are induced, more energy is needed to advance the crack, and crack blunting occurs.

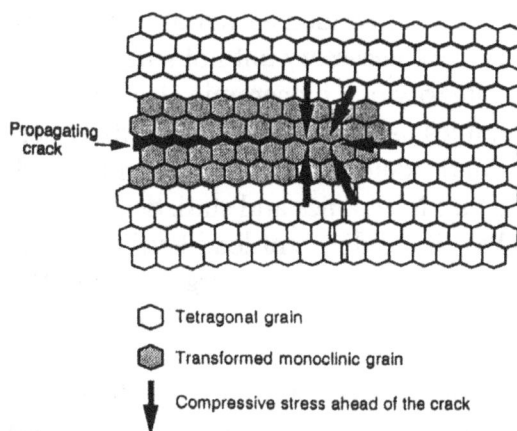

Propagating crack

○ Tetragonal grain

⬡ Transformed monoclinic grain

↓ Compressive stress ahead of the crack

Figure: Schematic of microstructure in yttrium partially stabilized zirconia (YPSZ) bioceramic undergoing transformation toughening at a crack tip.

The wear rate of YPSZ on UHMWPE can be five times less than the wear rate of alumina on UHMWPE, depending on experimental conditions. Wear resistance is a function of grain size, surface roughness, and residual compressive stresses induced by the phase transformation. The increased mechanical properties may allow for smaller-diameter femoral heads to be used in comparison with alumina.

Partially stabilized zirconia is typically shaped by cold isostatic pressing and then densified by sintering. Sintering may be performed with or without a subsequent hot isostatic pressing (HIP-ing) cycle. The material is usually presintered until approximately 95 percent dense and then HIP-ed to remove residual porosity. Sintering can be performed without inducing grain growth, and final grain sizes can be less than 1 μm.

Critical Properties of Bioinert Ceramics

In addition to wear resistance and minimal biological response, other properties of bioinert ceramics important for their long-term efficacy are stiffness, strength, and toughness. Stiffness represents one gauge of the mechanical interaction between an implant and its surrounding tissue; it is one determinant of the stress magnitude and distribution in the biomaterial as well as the tissue, and it also dictates the efficacy of stress transfer and potential for stress shielding. Although the effect of biomaterial stiffness has never been truly assessed in a functionally loaded prosthesis under controlled conditions in which stiffness was the only variable, it is generally acknowledged that stiffness is an important design parameter.

Load-bearing biomaterials must also be conservatively designed to ensure that they maintain their structural integrity, i.e., designed to be fail-safe at stresses above peak in-service stresses for a lifetime greater than the expected service life of the prosthesis. Thus the static (tensile, compressive, and flexural strength), dynamic (high-cycle fatigue), and toughness properties of ceramics in physiological media under a multitude of loading conditions and rates must be well characterized.

Although the types of data recommended earlier are an important aspect of any bioceramic database, these data are necessary but not sufficient input for designing bioceramics. The mechanical integrity of a bioceramic also depends on its processing, size, and shape. Failure of ceramics usually initiates at a critical defect at a stress level that depends on the geometry of the defect. To account for these variables and minimize the probability of failure, fracture mechanics and statistical distributions are recommended to predict failure probability at different load levels. Statistical methods are useful to account for scatter in properties, which is largely due to the random nature of the defects in these brittle materials. Ceramics are well suited for applying these fracture mechanics concepts because of the validity of linear elastic fracture mechanics for this class of materials. Crack growth behavior may be predicted based on stresses and the size and shape of existing flaws. Through the use of a proof test, the maximum allowable flaw sizes, minimum failure loads, and minimum service life can be predicted for a given set of conditions.

Bioactive Ceramics

The concept of bioactivity was introduced with respect to bioactive glasses via the following hypothesis: the biocompatibility of an implant material is optimal if the material elicits the formation of normal tissues at its surface and in addition if it establishes a contiguous interface capable of supporting the loads that normally occur at the site of implantation. Under appropriate conditions, three classes of ceramics may fulfill these requirements: bioactive glasses and glass ceramics, calcium phosphate ceramics, and composites of these glasses and ceramics. Additionally, incorporation of inductive factors into each of these classes may enhance bioactivity. Collectively, these different classes of materials/biological constituents are used clinically and experimentally in a wide variety of applications, including bulk implants (surface-active), coatings on metallic or ceramic implants (surface-active), permanent bone augmentation devices/ scaffold materials (surface-active), temporary tissue engineering devices (surface- or bulk-active), fillers such as in cements (surface- or bulk-active), and drug-delivery vehicles (bulk-active).

It is important to reemphasize that the nature of the biomaterial-tissue interface and the reactions (e.g., ion exchange) at the ceramic surface and in the tissues dictate the resulting mechanical, chemical, physical, and biological processes that occur. In general, four factors determine the long- term effect of bioactive ceramic implants: (1) the site of implantation, (2) tissue trauma, (3) the bulk and surface properties of the material, and (4) the relative motion at the implant-tissue interface. For resorbable materials, additional design requirements include the following: the strength/stability of the material-tissue interface needs to be maintained during the period of degradation and replacement by host tissue; material resorption and tissue repair/ regeneration rates should be matched; and the resorbable material should consist only of metabolically acceptable species.

Bioactive Glasses and Glass Ceramics

Bioactive glasses were first developed by Hench, who synthesized several glasses containing mixtures of silica, phosphate, calcia, and soda. These materials are used as bulk implants, coatings on metallic or ceramic implants, and scaffolds for guiding biological therapies.

Chemical reactions are limited to the surface (~300 to 500 µm) of the glass, and bulk properties are not affected by surface reactivity. The degree of activity and physiological response depends on the chemical composition of the glass and may vary by over an order of magnitude. For example, the substitution of CaF for CaO decreases the solubility of the glass, whereas the addition of B_2O_3 increases the solubility of the glass.

Ceravital, a variation of Bioglass, is a glass ceramic. The material is first quench-melted to form a glass and then heat-treated to form nuclei for crystal growth and subsequent transformation from a glass to a ceramic. Compared with Bioglass, Ceravital has a different alkali oxide concentration— small amounts of alkaline oxides are added to control dissolution rates but the physiological response of both these glasses is similar. It is hypothesized that the general biologic response to both glasses is the nucleation of hydroxyapatite crystals at the implant surface within an ordered collagen matrix, followed by the formation of mineralized bone.

A glass ceramic containing crystalline oxyapatite and fluorapatite [$Ca_{10}(PO_4)_6(O,F_2)$] and β Wollastonite (SiO_2-CaO) in a MgO-CaO-SiO_2 glassy matrix (denoted glass-ceramic A-W) represents a third bioactive glass. This material is formed by heating a glass powder compact, having a composition at 1050°C. A-W glass ceramic bonds to living bone through a thin calcium- and phosphorus-rich layer that is formed at the surface of the glass ceramic. If the physiological environment is correctly simulated in terms of ion concentration, pH, and temperature, this layer consists of small carbonated hydroxyapatite crystallites with a defective structure, and the composition and structural characteristics are similar to those of bone.

The physical/chemical basis for glass and glass-ceramic interfacing with the biologic milieu is as follows: ceramics are susceptible to surface changes in an aqueous medium. Lower-valence ions tend to segregate to surfaces and grain boundaries, leading to concentration gradients and ion exchange. These reactions depend on the local pH and reactive cellular constituents. It is important to note that these reactions can be either biologically beneficial or adverse and therefore must be well controlled and characterized as a function of microstructure and surface state.

Table: Composition (Weight Percent) of Bioactive Glasses and Glass Ceramics

Material	45S5 Bioglass	45S5-F Bioglass	45S5-B5 Bioglass	52S4.6 Bioglass	Ceravital	Stabilized Ceravital	A-W glass ceramic
SiO_2	45.0	45.0	45.0	52.0	40–50	40–50	34.2
P_2O_5	6.0	6.0	6.0	6.0	10–15	7.5–12.0	16.3
CaO	24.5	12.3	24.5	21.0	30–35	25–30	44.9
Na_2O	24.5	24.5	24.5	21.0	5–10	3.5–7.5	—
B_2O_3	—	—	5.0	—	—	—	—
CaF_2	—	12.3	—	—	—	—	0.5
K_2O	—	—	—	—	0.5–3.0	0.5–2.0	—
MgO	—	—	—	—	2.5–5.0	1.0–2.5	4.6
Al_2O_3	—	—	—	—	—	5.0–15.0	—
TiO_2	—	—	—	—	—	1.0–5.0	—
Ta_2O_5	—	—	—	—	—	5.0–15.0	—

When placed in a physiological medium, bioactive glasses leach Na^+ ions and subsequently also K+, Ca^{2+}, P^{5+}, Si^{4+}, and SiOH species. These ionic species are replaced with H_3O^+ ions from the medium through an ion-exchange reaction that produces a silica-rich gel surface layer. In an in vitro setting at least, the depletion of H^+/H_3O^+ ions in solution causes a pH increase, which further enhances glass dissolution. With increasing time of exposure to the medium, the highsurface-area silica-rich surface gel chelates calcium and phosphate ions, and a Ca-P-rich amorphous apatite layer forms on top of the silica-rich layer. This Ca-P-rich layer may form after as little as 1 hour in physiological solution. The amorphous Ca-P layer eventually crystallizes, and CO_3^{2-} substitutes for OH⁻ in the apatite lattice, leading to the formation of a carbonated apatite layer. Depending on animal species, anatomic site, and time of implantation, steady-state thickness of the Ca-P-rich and Si-rich zones can range from 30 to 70 μm and 60 to 230 um respectively.

In parallel with these physical/chemical-mediated reactions, in an in vivo setting, proteins adsorb/ desorb from the silica gel and carbonated layers. The bioactive surface and subsequent preferential protein adsorption that can occur can enhance attachment, differentiation, and proliferation of osteoblasts and secretion of the cells' own extracellular matrix. Crystallization of carbonated apatite within an ordered collagen matrix leads to an interfacial bond.

The overall rate of change of the glass surface R may be quantified as the sum of the reaction rates of each stage of the reaction:

$$R = k_1 t^{0.5} - k_2 t^{1.0} + k_3 t^{1.0} + k_4 t^{y} + k_5 t^{z}$$

where k is the rate constant for each stage and represents, respectively, the rate of exchange between alkali cations in glass and H^+/H_3O^+ in solution (k_1), interfacial SiO2 network dissolution (k_2), repolymerization of SiO_2 (k_3), carbonate precipitation and growth (k_4), and other precipitation reactions (k_5). Using these rates, the following design criterion may be established: The kinetics of each stage, especially stage 4, should match the rate of biomineralization in vivo. For $R \gg$ in vivo rates, resorption will occur, whereas if $\ll R$ in vivo rates, the glass will be nonbioactive .

The degree of activity and physiological response (e.g., rate of formation of the Ca-P surface and ultimate glass-tissue bond) therefore depends on the composition of the glass as well as on time and is mediated by the material, the solution, and the cell. The reactivity and rate of bond formation depend on composition and can be expressed by the ratio of the network former to the network modifier: $SiO_2 / (CaO + Na_2O + K_2O)$. The higher this ratio is, the less soluble is the glass and the slower is the rate of bone formation. Inspection of a $SiO_2 - Na_2O - CaO$ ternary diagram enables a quantitative association between composition and biological response (Hench, 1996). In general, the ternary diagram may be divided into three zones of biological interest: zone A, bioactive bone bonding [glasses are characterized by CaO/P_2O_5 ratios > 5 and $SiO_2/(CaO + Na_2O)$ ratios < 2]; zone B, nearly inert [bone bonding does not occur (only fibrous tissue formation occurs at the surface) because the SiO_2 content is too high and reactivity is too low; these high-SiO_2 glasses develop only a surface hydration layer or too dense a silica-rich layer to enable further dissolution and ion exchange]; and zone C, resorbable glasses (no bone bonding occurs because reactivity is too high and SiO_2 undergoes rapid selective alkali ion exchange with protons or H_3O^+, leading to a thick but porous unprotected SiO_2-rich film that dissociates at a high rate).

The level of bioactivity has been related to the physiological process of bone formation via an index of bioactivity I_B that is related to the amount of time it takes for 50 percent of the interface to be bonded:

$$I_B = 100 / t_{0.5BB}$$

The compositional dependence of the biological response may therefore be understood by viewing iso-IB contours superposed onto the ternary diagram. The cohesion strength of the glass-tissue interface will be a function of the surface area, thickness, and stiffness of the inerfacial zone and is optimum for $I_B \sim 4$.

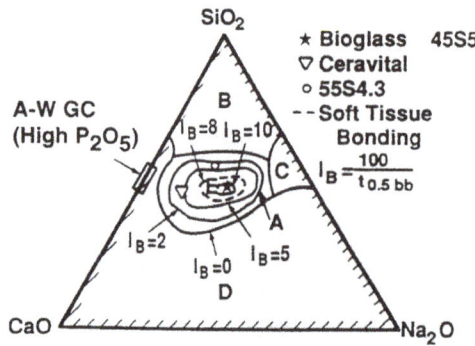

Figure: Ternary diagram

Ternary diagram (SiO_2 - Na_2O- CaO, at fixed 6 percent P_2O_5 SiO_2 -Na_2 O-CaO, at fixed 6 percent P_2O_5) showing the compositional dependence (in weight percent) of bone bonding and fibrous tissue bonding to the surfaces of bioactive glasses and glass ceramics: zone A, bioactive bone bonding ceramics; zone B, nearly inert ceramics (bone bonding does not occur at the ceramic surface; only fibrous tissue formation occurs); zone C, resorbable ceramics (no bone bonding occurs because reactivity is too high). I_B = index of bioactivity for bioceramics in zone A.

Calcium-Phosphate Ceramics

Calcium phosphate ceramics are ceramics with varying calcium-to-phosphate ratios. Among them, the apatite ceramics, defined by the chemical formula $M_{10}(XO_4)_6 Z_2$, have been studied most. The apatites form a range of solid solutions as a result of ionic substitution at the M^{2+}, XO_4^{3-}, or Z- sites. In general, apatites are nonstoichiometric and contain less than 10 mol of M^{2+} ions, less than 2 mol of Z- ions, and exactly 6 mol of XO_4^{3-} ions. The M^{2+} species is typically a bivalent metallic cation, such as Ca^{2+}, Sr^{2+}, Ba^{2+}, Pb^{2+}, or Cd^{2+}. The XO_4^{3-} species is typically one of the following trivalent anions: AsO_4^{3-}, VO_4^{3-}, CrO_4^{3-}, or MnO_4^{3-}. The monovalent Z- ions are usually F^- , OH^- , Br^-.

More complex ionic structures may also exist. For example, replacing the two monovalent Z- ions with a bivalent ion, such as CO_3^{2-}, results in the preservation of charge neutrality, but one anionic position becomes vacant. Similarly, the M^{2+} positions may also have vacancies. In this case, charge neutrality is maintained by vacancies at the Z- positions or by substitution of some trivalent ions with bivalent ions.

The most common apatite used in medicine and dentistry is hydroxyapatite (HA), a material with a hexagonal crystal lattice; an ideal chemical formula, i.e., $Ca_{10}\left(PO_4\right)_6\left(OH\right)_2$; ideal weight percents of 39.9 percent Ca, 18.5 percent P, and 3.38 percent OH; and an ideal calcium-phosphate ratio of 1.67. The crystal structure and crystallization behavior of HA is strongly dependent on the substitutional nature of the ionic species.

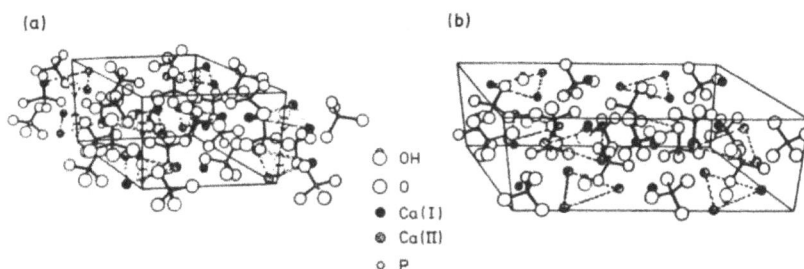

Figure: Schematic of hydroxyapatite crystal structure: (a) hexagonal; (b) monoclinic.

The impetus for using synthetic HA as a biomaterial stems from the perceived advantage of using a material similar to the mineral phase in bone and teeth for replacing these materials. Better tissue bonding is therefore expected. Additional potential advantages of bioactive ceramics include low thermal and electrical conductivity, elastic properties similar to those of bone, control of in vivo degradation rates through control of material properties, and the ceramic functioning as a barrier when coated onto a metal substrate.

Two aspects of the crystal chemistry of natural and synthetic apatites need to be recognized. First, the HA in bone is nonstoichiometric, has a Ca/P ratio of less than 1.67, and contains carbonate ions, sodium, magnesium, fluorine, and chlorine (Posner, 1985a). Second, most synthetic hydroxyapatites actually contain substitutions for the phosphate and/or hydroxyl groups and vary from the ideal stoichiometry and Ca/P ratios. Oxyhydroxyapatite [Ca10(PO4)6O], α-tricalcium phosphate $\left(\alpha - TCP\right)$, β tricalcium phosphate $\left(\beta - TCP\right)$ or β - Whitlockite $\left[Ca_3\left(PO_4\right)_2\right]$, tetracalcium phosphate $\left(Ca_4P_2O_9\right)$, and octocalcium phosphate $\left[Ca_8\left(HPO_4\right)_2\left(PO_4\right)_4\cdot5H_2O\right]$ have all been detected via x-ray diffraction (XRD), Fourier transform infrared spectroscopy (FTIR), and chemical analyses. These compounds are not apatites per se since the crystal structure differs from that of actual apatite.

Numerous processing techniques have been developed for producing synthetic apatites, including hydrolysis, hydrothermal synthesis and exchange, sol-gel techniques, wet chemistry, and conversion of natural bone and coral. Because of the variability in processing strategies, it is critical to appreciate that differences in the structure, chemistry, and composition of apatites arise from differences in material processing techniques, time, temperature, and atmosphere. Understanding the processing composition structure processing synergy for calcium phosphates is therefore critical to understanding the in vivo function of these materials.

As stoichiometric HA is heated from room temperature, it may become dehydrated. Between 25 and 200°C, adsorbed water is reversibly lost. Between 200 and 400°C, lattice-bound water (from H_2O or $2HPO_4^{2-}$ substituting OH^- or PO_4^{3-} ions) is irreversibly lost, causing a contraction of the crystal lattice. Lattice water is only present when synthetic apatite is prepared from an aqueous system. At temperatures greater than 850°C, a reversible weight loss occurs, indicating another reversible dehydration reaction. Should pyrolysis occur, an oxyhydroxyapatite forms. Above 1050°C, HA may decompose into β-TCP and tetracalcium phosphate, by the following reaction: $Ca_{10}(PO_4)_6(OH)_2 \rightarrow 2\beta Ca_3(PO_4)_2 + Ca_4P_2O_9 + H_2O$. At temperatures above 1350°C, β-TCP transforms into α-TCP, which is retained on cooling. Analogous reactions occur with nonstoichiometric hydroxyapatite, but the reaction products differ as a function of the Ca/P ratio.

The dissolution behavior of HA in an aqueous medium and subsequent biological reactions also depend on the chemical composition of the crystal. Ion exchange occurring at the apatite surface depends on (1) the rate of formation and dissolution of the various phases, (2) the powder-weight-toliquid-volume ratio, (3) pH, (4) specific surface area, (5) crystal defects, impurities, and vacancies, and (6) substitutional ions.

The general mechanism of biological bonding to calcium phosphates is as follows. Differentiated osteoblasts secrete a mineralized matrix at the ceramic surface, resulting in a narrow, amorphous electron-dense band approximately 3 to 5 μm thick. Collagen bundles form between this zone and the cells. Bone mineral crystals nucleate within this amorphous zone, first in the form of an octocalcium phosphate precursor phase, and, ultimately they undergo a conversion to HA. As the healing site matures, the bonding zone shrinks to approximately 0.05 to 0.2 μm, and bone attaches through a thin epitaxial bonding layer to the bulk implant as the growing bone crystals align with the apatite crystals of material.

Calcium-phosphate-based bioceramics have also been used as coatings on dense implants and porous surface layers to accelerate and enhance fixation of a substrate biomaterial to tissue. Results of these studies vary with respect to bond strength, solubility, and overall in vivo function, suggesting a window of material variability in parallel with a window of biologic variability.

Numerous processing techniques are used to deposit and bond Ca-P powders to substrates, including plasma and thermal spraying, ion-beam and other sputter-deposition techniques, electrophoretic deposition, sintering, sol-gel techniques, pulsed laser deposition, and chemical vapor deposition.

During plasma spraying, powder is sprayed onto a metal core. Plasma temperatures as high as 10,000 °C can be reached. The ceramic particles form a loosely bonded coating on impact. Due to the rapid cooling of the particles, the temperature of the metal remains low, and the structure and properties of the bulk metal remain unchanged.

However, porosity and phase changes are induced in the ceramic. For example, mixtures of HA, TCP, and tetracalcium phosphate evolve as a result of plasma spraying nominally pure HA.

During sputter deposition, a beam (ion) sputters off atoms from a target to form a thin coating on a substrate. During electrophoretic deposition, the calcium-phosphate ceramic (CPC) is precipitated out of suspension onto a substrate. An advantage of this technique, as well as low-temperature sol-gel techniques, is that it is more conducive to coating the internal surfaces of a porous substrate. Both sintering and electrophoretic deposition of hydroxyapatite onto titanium result in an interfacial layer rich in Ti and P. The interfacial zone has a different composition from that of the bulk Ca-P coating.

The different structures and compositions of Ca-P coatings resulting from different processing modulate the subsequent biological reactions. For example, increased Ca/P ratios, fluorine and carbonate contents, and degree of crystallinity all lead to greater stability of the biological precipitate. In general, calcium phosphates with Ca/P ratios in the range 1.5 to 1.67 (tricalcium phosphate and HA, respectively) yield the most beneficial tissue response. Given the range of chemical compositions available in bioactive ceramics and the resulting fact that pure HA is used rarely, the broader term calcium-phosphate ceramics has been proposed in lieu of the more specific term hydroxyapatite. Each individual CPC is defined by its own unique set of chemical and physical properties.

Bioactive Ceramic Composites

Bioactive ceramics typically exhibit low strength and toughness. The reason for the mechanical deficiency is that the design requirement of bioactivity supersedes any mechanical property requirement, and as a result, mechanical properties are restricted. Bioceramic composites therefore have been synthesized as a means of creating a material with superior properties to that of the individual constituents. Three separate design objectives are used as criteria for developing bioceramic composites: (1) use the beneficial biological response to bioceramics and reinforce the ceramic with a second phase to strengthen the ceramic, (2) use bioceramic materials as the second phase to achieve desirable strengths and stiffnesses, and (3) synthesize scaffold materials for tissue (re)generation.

Bioactive glass composites have been synthesized via thermal treatments that create a second phase. By altering the firing temperature and composition of the bioactive glasses, stable multiphase bioactive glass composites have been produced. Adding oxyapatite, fluorapatite, β-Wollastonite, and/or β-Whitlockite results in bending strengths two to five times greater than that of unreinforced bioactive glasses. Calcium phosphates have been strengthened via incorporation of glasses, alumina, and zirconia.

Critical Properties of Bioactive Ceramics

Important issues in bioactive ceramics research and development still include characterization of the processing-composition-structure-property synergy, characterization of in vivo function, and establishing the relationship between in vitro and in vivo function. Parameters important to understanding and improving the ceramic-tissue bond and reactions at the ceramic surface and in the tissues have been outlined:

(1) Characterization of surface activity, including surface analysis, biochemistry, and ion transport,

(2) Physical chemistry, pertaining to strength and degradation, stability of the tissue-ceramic interface, and tissue resorption, and

(3) Biomechanics, as related to strength, stiffness, design, wear, and tissue remodeling. It is essential to note that these properties are time-dependent and therefore must be characterized as a function of loading and environmental history.

Specific physicochemical properties that are important to characterize and relate to in vitro and in vivo biologic response include powder particle size and shape; pore size, shape, and distribution; specific surface area; phases present; crystal structure and size; grain size; density; coating thickness; hardness; and surface roughness.

Starting powders may be identified for their particle size, shape, and distribution via sifting techniques or more quantitative stereological imaging techniques. Pore size, shape, and distribution, important properties with respect to strength and bioreactivity, also may be quantified via stereological methods and/or scanning electron microscopy (SEM). Specific surface area, important in understanding the dissolution and precipitation reactions at the ceramic-fluid interface, may be characterized by the Brunnauer, Emmet, and Teller (BET) technique.

Phase identification may be accomplished via XRD. FTIR is recommended as a complementary technique because it allows identification of phase amounts and structures not readily detectable with XRD. Grain sizes may be determined through optical microscopy, SEM, or transmission electron microscopy (TEM), depending on the order of the grain size. Additionally, TEM is useful to characterize second phases, crystal structure, and lattice imperfections. Auger electron spectroscopy (AES) and x-ray photoelectron spectroscopy (XPS) may also be utilized to determine surface and interfacial compositions. Chemical stability and surface activity may be analyzed via XPS and measurements of ionic fluxes and zeta potentials. It is assumed that two different pathways of activity exist: solution and cell-mediated.

An additional parameter that should be considered in evaluating chemical stability and surface activity of bioceramics is the simulated in vivo environment. Factors such as the type and concentration of electrolytes in solution and the presence of proteins or cells may influence in vitro immersion results. For example, in a study on glass-ceramic A-W that can be generalized to other bioceramics, a solution with constituents, concentrations, and pH equivalent to human plasma most accurately reproduces in vivo surface structural changes, whereas more standard buffers do not reproduce these changes.

The physiologic response at a biomaterial-tissue interface depends on both the implant and the tissue. Therefore, analyses of both these constituents must be well posed: the implant surface must be analyzed, and the species released into the environment and tissues also must be determined. Analysis can be accomplished with solution chemical methods, such as atomic absorption spectroscopy; physical methods, such as thin-film XRD, electron microprobe analysis (BMP), energy dispersive xray analysis (EDXA), and FTIR; and surf ace-sensitive methods, such as AES, XPS, and secondary ions mass spectroscopy (SIMS). The type of loading is also important in analyzing bonebonding behavior. The integrity of the implant-tissue interface is strongly dependent on the specific nature of the loading pattern since loading may alter the chemical and mechanical behavior of the interface.

The major factor limiting expanded use of bioactive ceramics is their low tensile strength and fracture toughness. Their use in bulk form is therefore limited to functions in which only compressive loads are applied. To use ceramics as self-standing implants that are able to withstand tensile stresses is a primary engineering design objective. Four general approaches have been used to achieve this objective:

(1) Use of the bioactive ceramic as a coating on a metal or ceramic substrate,

(2) Strengthening of the ceramic, such as via crystallization of glass,

(3) Use of fracture mechanics as a design approach, and

(4) reinforcing of the ceramic with a second phase.

No matter which of these four strategies is used, the resulting bioactive ceramic must be stable, both chemically and mechanically, until it fulfills its intended function(s). It should be noted, however, that the specific properties needed depend on the specific application. For example, if a smooth total hip prosthesis is to be fixed by coating the metal stem with a CPC coating, then the ceramic-metal bond must remain intact throughout the service life of the prosthesis. However, if the CPC coating is used on a porous-coated prosthesis with the intent of accelerating ingrowth into the pores of the metal, then the ceramic-metal bond need only be stable until tissue ingrowth is achieved.

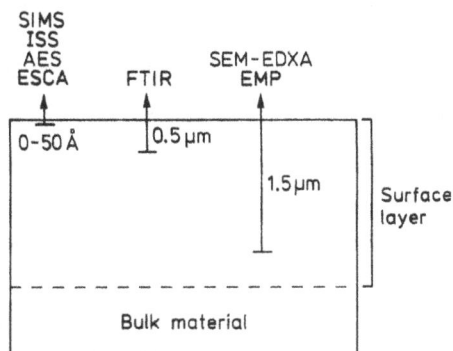

Figure: Schematic of sampling depths for different surface analysis techniques used to characterize bioceramics.

Applications

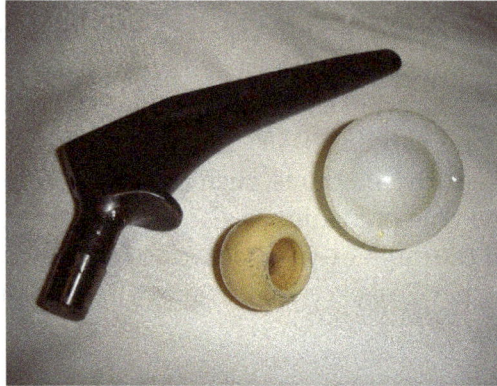

A titanium hip prosthesis, with a ceramic head and polyethylene acetabular cup

Ceramics are now commonly used in the medical fields as dental and bone implants. Surgical cermets are used regularly. Joint replacements are commonly coated with bioceramic materials to reduce wear and inflammatory response. Other examples of medical uses for bioceramics are in pacemakers, kidney dialysis machines, and respirators. The global demand on medical ceramics and ceramic components was about U.S. $9.8 billion in 2010. It was forecast to have an annual growth of 6 to 7 percent in the following years, with world market value predicted to increase to U.S. $15.3 billion by 2015 and reach U.S. $18.5 billion by 2018.

Mechanical Properties and Composition

Bioceramics are meant to be used in extracorporeal circulation systems (dialysis for example) or engineered bioreactors; however, they›re most common as implants. Ceramics show numerous applications as biomaterials due to their physico-chemical properties. They have the advantage of being inert in the human body, and their hardness and resistance to abrasion makes them useful for bones and teeth replacement. Some ceramics also have excellent resistance to friction, making them useful as replacement materials for malfunctioning joints. Properties such as appearance and electrical insulation are also a concern for specific biomedical applications.

Some bioceramics incorporate alumina (Al_2O_3) as their lifespan is longer than that of the patient's. The material can be used in inner ear ossicles, ocular prostheses, electrical insulation for pacemakers, catheter orifices and in numerous prototypes of implantable systems such as cardiac pumps.

Aluminosilicates are commonly used in dental prostheses, pure or in ceramic-polymer composites. The ceramic-polymer composites are a potential way to filling of cavities replacing amalgams suspected to have toxic effects. The aluminosilicates also have a glassy structure. Contrary to artificial teeth in resin, the colour of tooth ceramic remains stable Zirconia doped with yttrium oxide has been proposed as a substitute for alumina for osteoarticular prostheses. The main advantages are greater failure strength, and a good resistance to fatigue.

Vitreous carbon is also used as it is light, resistant to wear, and compatible with blood. It is mostly used in cardiac valve replacement. Diamond can be used for the same application, but in coating form.

Calcium phosphate-based ceramics constitute, at present, the preferred bone substitute in orthopaedic and maxillofacial surgery. They are similar to the mineral phase of the bone in structure and/or chemical composition. The material is typically porous, which provide a good bone-implant interface due to the increase of surface area that encourages cell colonisation and revascularisation. Additionally, it has lower mechanical strength compared to bone, making highly porous implants very delicate. Since Young's modulus of ceramics is generally much higher than that of the bone tissue, the implant can cause mechanical stresses at the bone interface. Calcium phosphates usually found in bioceramics include hydroxyapatite (HAP) $Ca_{10}(PO_4)_6(OH)_2$; tricalcium phosphate β (β TCP): $Ca_3(PO_4)_2$; and mixtures of HAP and β TCP.

Table: Bioceramics Applications

Devices	Function	Biomaterial
Artificial total hip, knee, shoulder, elbow, wrist	Reconstruct arthritic or fractured joints	High-density alumina, metal bioglass coatings
Bone plates, screws, wires	Repair fractures	Bioglass-metal fibre composite, Polysulphone-carbon fibre composite
Intramedullary nails	Align fractures	Bioglass-metal fibre composite, Polysulphone-carbon fibre composite
Harrington rods	Correct chronic spinal curvature	Bioglass-metal fibre composite, Polysulphone-carbon fibre composite
Permanently implanted artificial limbs	Replace missing extremities	Bioglass-metal fibre composite, Polysulphone-carbon fibre composite
Vertebrae Spacers and extensors	Correct congenital deformity	Al_2O_3
Spinal fusion	Immobilise vertebrae to protect spinal cord	Bioglass
Alveolar bone replacements, mandibular reconstruction	Restore the alveolar ridge to improve denture fit	Polytetra fluro ethylene (PTFE) - carbon composite, Porous Al_2O_3, Bioglass, dense-apatite
End osseous tooth replacement implants	Replace diseased, damaged or loosened teeth	Al_2O_3, Bioglass, dense hydroxyapatite, vitreous carbon
Orthodontic anchors	Provide posts for stress application required to change deformities	Bioglass-coated Al_2O_3, Bioglass coated vitallium

Table: Mechanical Properties of Ceramic Biomaterials

Material	Young's Modulus (GPa)	Compressive Strength (MPa)	Bond strength (GPa)	Hardness	Density (g/cm³)
Inert Al_2O_3	380	4000	300-400	2000-3000(HV)	>3.9
ZrO_2 (PS)	150-200	2000	200-500	1000-3000(HV)	≈6.0
Graphite	20-25	138	NA	NA	1.5-1.9
(LTI)Pyrolitic Carbon	17-28	900	270-500	NA	1.7-2.2
Vitreous Carbon	24-31	172	70-207	150-200(DPH)	1.4-1.6
Bioactive HAP	73-117	600	120	350	3.1
Bioglass	≈75	1000	50	NA	2.5
AW Glass Ceramic	118	1080	215	680	2.8
Bone	3-30	130-180	60-160	NA	NA

Multipurpose

A number of implanted ceramics have not actually been designed for specific biomedical applications. However, they manage to find their way into different implantable systems because of their properties and their good biocompatibility. Among these ceramics, we can cite silicon carbide, titanium nitrides and carbides, and boron nitride. TiN has been suggested as the friction surface in hip prostheses. While cell culture tests show a good biocompatibility, the analysis of implants shows significant wear, related to a delaminating of the TiN layer. Silicon carbide is another modern-day ceramic which seems to provide good biocompatibility and can be used in bone implants.

Specific use

In addition to being used for their traditional properties, bioactive ceramics have seen specific use for due to their biological activity. Calcium phosphates, oxides, and hydroxides are common examples. Other natural materials — generally of animal origin — such as bioglass and other composites feature a combination of mineral-organic composite materials such as HAP, alumina, or titanium dioxide with the biocompatible polymers (polymethylmethacrylate): PMMA, poly(L-lactic) acid: PLLA, poly(ethylene). Composites can be differentiated as bioresorbable or non-bioresorbable, with the latter being the result of the combination of a non-bioresorbable calcium phosphate (HAP) with a non-bioresorbable polymer (PMMA, PE). These materials may become more widespread in the future, on account of the many combination possibilities and their aptitude at combining a biological activity with mechanical properties similar to those of the bone.

Biocompatibility

Bioceramics' properties of being anticorrosive, biocompatible, and aesthetic make them quite suitable for medical usage. Zirconia ceramic has bioinertness and non-cytotoxicity.

Carbon is another alternative with similar mechanical properties to bone, and it also features blood compatibility, no tissue reaction, and non-toxicity to cells. None of the three bioinert ceramics exhibit bonding with the bone. However, bioactivity of bioinert ceramics can be achieved by forming composites with bioactive ceramics. Bioglass and glass ceramics are nontoxic and chemically bond to bone. Glass ceramics elicit osteoinductive properties, while calcium phosphate ceramics also exhibit non-toxicity to tissues and bioresorption. The ceramic particulate reinforcement has led to the choice of more materials for implant applications that include ceramic/ceramic, ceramic/polymer, and ceramic/metal composites. Among these composites ceramic/polymer composites have been found to release toxic elements into the surrounding tissues. Metals face corrosion related problems, and ceramic coatings on metallic implants degrade over time during lengthy applications. Ceramic/ceramic composites enjoy superiority due to similarity to bone minerals, exhibiting biocompatibility and a readiness to be shaped. The biological activity of bioceramics has to be considered under various *in vitro* and *in vivo* studies. Performance needs must be considered in accordance with the particular site of implantation.

Processing

Technically, ceramics are composed of raw materials such as powders and natural or synthetic chemical additives, favoring either compaction (hot, cold or isostatic), setting (hydraulic or chemical), or accelerating sintering processes. According to the formulation and shaping process used, bioceramics can vary in density and porosity as cements, ceramic depositions, or ceramic composites.

A developing material processing technique based on the biomimetic processes aims to imitate natural and biological processes and offer the possibility of making bioceramics at ambient temperature rather than through conventional or hydrothermal processes [GRO 96]. The prospect of using these relatively low processing temperatures opens up possibilities for mineral organic combinations with improved biological properties through the addition of proteins and biologically active molecules (growth factors, antibiotics, anti-tumor agents, etc.). However, these materials have poor mechanical properties which can be improved, partially, by combining them with bonding proteins.

Commercial Usage

Common bioactive materials available commercially for clinical use include 45S5 bioactive glass, A/W bioactive glass ceramic, dense synthetic HA, and bioactive composites such as a polyethylene–HA mixture. All these materials form an interfacial bond with adjacent tissue.

High-purity alumina bioceramics are currently commercially available from various producers. U.K. manufacturer Morgan Advanced Ceramics (MAC) began manufacturing orthopaedic devices in 1985 and quickly became a recognised supplier of ceramic femoral heads for hip replacements. MAC Bioceramics has the longest clinical history for alumina ceramic materials, manufacturing HIP Vitox alumina since 1985. Some calcium-deficient phosphates with an apatite structure were thus commercialised as "tricalcium phosphate" even though they did not exhibit the expected crystalline structure of tricalcium phosphate.

Currently, numerous commercial products described as HA are available in various physical forms (e.g. granules, specially designed blocks for specific applications). HA/polymer composite (HA/polyethyelene, HAPEXTM) is also commercially available for ear implants, abrasives, and plasma-sprayed coating for orthopedic and dental implants.

Cell Encapsulation

Immobilization of living cells or other biomaterials in alginate gels is a well-known technology used in an increasing number of biomedical and industrial applications. Cells immobilized in alginate gels maintain good viability during long-term culture due to the mild environment of the gel network. In tissue engineering applications immobilized cells or tissue can be used as bioartificial organs as the alginate gel may function as a protective barrier towards physical stress and to avoid immunological reactions with the host. Such bioreactor systems, of which the entrapped cells are selected or manipulated to excrete therapeutic products, are currently being developed for the treatment of a variety of diseases like cancer and diabetes. For most uses, and in particular those involving immobilization of living cells, microcapsules are used. Smaller beads/capsules have the advantage of a higher surface to volume ratio allowing good transport of essential nutrients and are also less fragile. Diffusion limitations within larger beads may limit cellular metabolism as the lack of essential substances like oxygen supply to the interior of the beads may lead to cell death as a result of consumption from the surrounding cells. Therefore a good control of bead size and shape is crucial and should be carefully controlled. A suitable methodology for production of small beads under controlled conditions is therefore also necessary. The bead generators shown here are recommended alternatives for research use in the production of small spherical alginate beads containing biological materials and having a narrow size distribution.

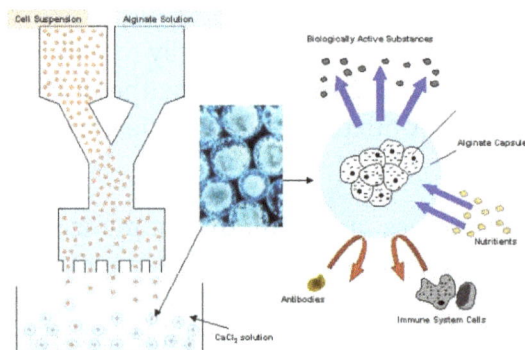

Commonly used principle for immobilization of cells in alginate beads for transplantation purposes. The beads may also be coated with other biopolymers and alginate for improved properties.

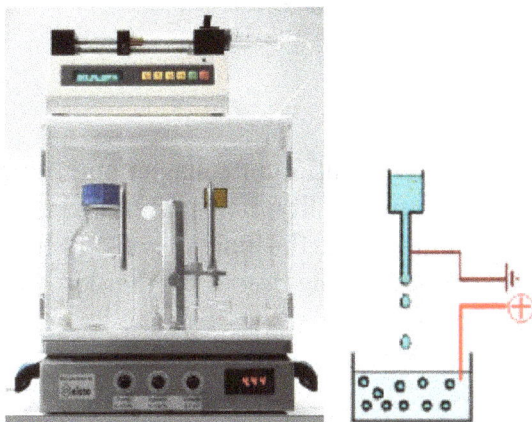

Small alginate beads with a narrow size distribution, ranging in size down to about 150 μm, can easily be manufactured by using the electrostatic bead generator. The basic principle of the instrument is the use of an electrostatic potential to pull the droplets from a nozzle tip. An electrostatic voltage of a few kV is set between the needle feeding the alginate solution and the gelling bath. The droplet size is also largely determined by selecting an appropriate nozzle size.

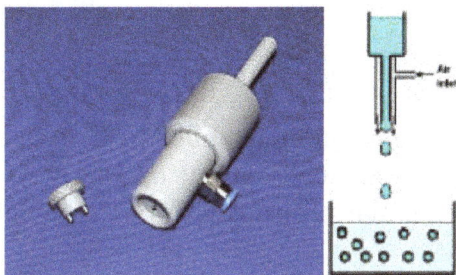

Small size alginate beads with a relatively narrow size distribution, ranging in size down to about 600 μm can be manufactured by the use of the coaxial bead generator. The basic principle of the instrument is the use of a coaxial air stream to pull droplets from a needle tip into a gelling bath. Bead size is controlled by adjusting the solution and gas- flow rates.

Collagen

Collagen, a major protein component of the ECM, provides support to tissues like skin, cartilage, bones, blood vessels and ligaments and is thus considered a model scaffold or matrix for tissue engineering due to its properties of biocompatibility, biodegradability and ability to promote cell binding. This ability allows chitosan to control distribution of cells inside the polymeric system. Thus, Type-I collagen obtained from animal tissues is now successfully being used commercially as tissue engineered biomaterial for multiple applications. Collagen has also been used in nerve repair and bladder engineering. Immunogenicity has limited the applications of collagen. Gelatin has been considered as an alternative for that reason.

Gelatin

Gelatin is prepared from the denaturation of collagen and many desirable properties such as biodegradability, biocompatibility, non-immunogenity in physiological environments, and easy processability make this polymer a good choice for tissue engineering applications. It is used in engineering tissues for the skin, bone and cartilage and is used commercially for skin replacements.

Chitosan

Chitosan is a polysaccharide composed of randomly distributed β-(1-4)-linked D-glucosamine (deacetylated unit) and N-acetyl-D-glucosamine (acetylated unit). It is derived from the N-deacetylation of chitin and has been used for several applications such as drug delivery, space-filling implants and in wound dressings. However, one drawback of this polymer is its weak mechanical properties and is thus often combined with other polymers such collagen to form a polymer with stronger mechanical properties for cell encapsulation applications.

Agarose

Agarose is a polysaccharide derived from seaweed used for nanoencapsulation of cells and the cell/agarose suspension can be modified to form microbeads by reducing the temperature during preparation. However, one drawback with the microbeads so obtained is the possibility of cellular protrusion through the polymeric matrix wall after formation of the capsules.

Cellulose Sulphate

Cellulose sulphate is derived from cotton and, once processed appropriately, can be used as a biocompatible base in which to suspend cells. When the poly-anionic cellulose sulphate solution is immersed in a second, poly-cationic solution (e.g. pDADMAC), a semi-permeable membrane is formed around the suspended cells as a result of gelation between the two poly-ions. Both mammalian cell lines and bacterial cells remain viable and continue to replicate within the capsule membrane in order to fill-out the capsule. As such, in contrast to some other encapsulation materials, the capsules can be used to grow cells and act as such like a mini-bioreactor. The biocompatible nature of the material has been demonstrated by observation during studies using the cell-filled capsules themselves for implantation as well as isolated capsule material. Capsules formed from cellulose sulphate have been successfully used, showing safety and efficacy, in clinical and pre-clinical trials in both humans and animals, primarily as anti-cancer treatments, but also exploring possible uses for gene therapy or antibody therapies. Using cellulose sulphate it has been possible to manufacture encapsulated cells as a pharmaceutical product at large scale and fulfilling Good Manufacturing Process (cGMP) standards. This was achieved by the company Austrianova in 2007.

Biocompatibility

The use of an ideal high quality biomaterial with the inherent properties of biocompatibility is the most crucial factor that governs the long term efficiency of this technology. An ideal biomaterial for cell encapsulation should be one that is totally biocompatible, does not trigger an immune response in the host and does not interfere with cell homeostasis so as to ensure high cell viability. However, one major limitation has been the inability to reproduce the different biomaterials and the requirements to obtain a better understanding of the chemistry and biofunctionality of the biomaterials and the microencapsulation system. Several studies demonstrate that surface modification of these cell containing microparticles allows control over the growth and cellular differentiation. of the encapsulated cells.

One study proposed the use of zeta potential which measures the electric charge of the microcapsule as a means to predict the interfacial reaction between microcapsule and the surrounding tissue and in turn the biocompatibility of the delivery system.

Microcapsule Permeability

A fundamental criterion that must be established while developing any device with a semi-permeable membrane is to adjust the permeability of the device in terms of entry and exit of molecules. It is essential that the cell microcapsule is designed with uniform thickness and should have a control over both the rate of molecules entering the capsule necessary for cell viability and the rate of therapeutic products and waste material exiting the capsule membrane. Immunoprotection of the loaded cell is the key issue that must be kept in mind while working on the permeability of the encapsulation membrane as not only immune cells but also antibodies and cytokines should be prevented entry into the microcapsule which in fact depends on the pore size of the biomembrane.

It has been shown that since different cell types have different metabolic requirements, thus depending on the cell type encapsulated in the membrane the permeability of the membrane has to be optimized. Several groups have been dedicated towards the study of membrane permeability of cell microcapsules and although the role of permeability of certain essential elements like oxygen has been demonstrated, the permeability requirements of each cell type are yet to be determined.

Sodium Citrate is used for degradation of alginate beads after encapsulation of cells. In order to determine viability of the cells or for further experimentation. Concentrations of approximately 25mM are used to dissolve the alginate spheres and the solution is spun down using a centrifuge so the sodium citrate can be removed and the cells can be collected.

Mechanical Strength and Durability

It is essential that the microcapsules have adequate membrane strength (mechanical stability) to endure physical and osmotic stress such as during the exchange of nutrients and waste products. The microcapsules should be strong enough and should not rupture on implantation as this could lead to an immune rejection of the encapsulated cells. For instance, in the case of xenotransplantation, a tighter more stable membrane would be required in comparison to allotransplantation. Also, while investigating the potential of using APA microcapsules loaded with bile salt hydrolase (BSH) overproducing active Lactobacillus plantarum 80 cells, in a simulated gastro intestinal tract model for oral delivery applications, the mechanical integrity and shape of the microcapsules was evaluated. It was shown that APA microcapsules could potentially be used in the oral delivery of live bacterial cells. However, further research proved that the GCAC microcapsules possess a higher mechanical stability as compared to APA microcapsules for oral delivery applications. Martoni was experimenting with bacteria-filled capsules that would be taken by mouth to reduce serum cholesterol. The capsules were pumped through a series of vessels simulating the human GI tract to determine how well the capsules would survive in the body. Extensive research into the mechanical properties of the biomaterial to be used for cell microencapsulation is necessary to determine the durability of the microcapsules during production and especially for in vivo applications where a sustained release of the therapeutic product over long durations is required. Van der Wijngaart grafted a solid, but permeable, shell around the cells to provide increased mechanical strength.

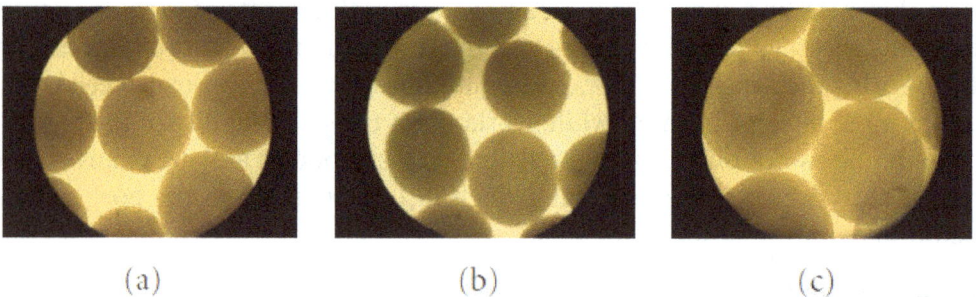

(a)   (b)   (c)

Illustration of the APA microcapsule integrity and morphological changes during simulated GI transit. (a) Pre-stomach transit. (b) Post-stomach transit (60 minutes). (c) Post-stomach (60 minutes) and intestinal (10-hour) transit. Microcapsule size: (a) 608 ± 36 μm (b) 544 ± 40 μm (c) 725 ± 55 μm.

Sodium Citrate is used for degradation of alginate beads after encapsulation of cells. In order to determine viability of the cells or for further experimentation. Concentrations of approximately 25mM are used to dissolve the alginate spheres and the solution is spun down using a centrifuge so the sodium citrate can be removed and the cells can be collected.

Methods for Testing Mechanical Properties of Microcapsules

- A Rheometer is a machine used to test
  - shear rate
  - shear strength
  - consistency coefficient
  - flow behavior index
- Viscometer - shear strength testing

Microcapsule Generation

Microfluidics

Droplet-based microfluidics can be used to generate microparticles with repeatable size:

- manipulation of alginate solution to allow microcapsules to be created.

Electrospraying Techniques

Eletrospraying is used to create alginate spheres by pumping an alginate solution through a needle. A source of high voltage usually provided by a clamp attached to the needle is used to generate an electric potential with the alginate falling from the needle tip into a solution that contains a ground. Calcium chloride is used as cross linking solution in which the generated capsules drop into where they harden after approximately 30 minutes. Beads are formed from the needle due to charge and surface tension.

- Size dependency of the beads
- height alterations of device from needle to calcium chloride solution
- voltage alterations of clamp on the needle
- alginate concentration alterations

Microcapsule Size

The diameter of the microcapsules is an important factor that influences both the immune response towards the cell microcapsules as well as the mass transport across the capsule membrane. Studies show that the cellular response to smaller capsules is much lesser as compared to larger capsules and in general the diameter of the cell loaded microcapsules should be between 350-450 μm so as to enable effective diffusion across the semi-permeable membrane.

Cell Choice

The cell type chosen for this technique depends on the desired application of the cell microcapsules. The cells put into the capsules can be from the patient (autologous cells), from another donor (allogeneic cells) or from other species (xenogeneic cells). The use of autologous cells in microencapsulation therapy is limited by the availability of these cells and even though xenogeneic cells are easily accessible, danger of possible transmission of viruses, especially porcine endogenous retrovirus to the patient restricts their clinical application, and after much debate several groups have concluded that studies should involve the use of allogeneic instead of xenogeneic cells. Depending on the application, the cells can be genetically altered to express any required protein. However, enough research has to be carried out to validate the safety and stability of the expressed gene before these types of cells can be used.

This technology has not received approval for clinical trial because of the high immunogenicity of cells loaded in the capsules. They secrete cytokines and produce a severe inflammatory reaction at the implantation site around the capsules, in turn leading to a decrease in viability of the encapsulated cells. One promising approach being studied is the administration of anti-inflammatory drugs to reduce the immune response produced due to administration of the cell loaded microcapsules. Another approach which is now the focus of extensive research is the use of stem cells such as mesenchymal stem cells for long term cell microencapsulation and cell therapy applications in hopes of reducing the immune response in the patient after implantation. Another issue which compromises long term viability of the microencapsulated cells is the use of fast proliferating cell lines which eventually fill up the entire system and lead to decrease in the diffusion efficiency across the semi-permeable membrane of the capsule. A solution to this could be in the use of cell types such as myoblasts which do not proliferate after the microencapsulation procedure.

Non-Therapeutic Applications

Probiotics are increasingly being used in numerous dairy products such as ice cream, milk powders, yoghurts, frozen dairy desserts and cheese due to their important health benefits. But, low viability of probiotic bacteria in the food still remains a major hurdle. The pH, dissolved oxygen content, titratable acidity, storage temperature, species and strains of associative fermented dairy product organisms and concentration of lactic and acetic acids are some of the factors that greatly affect the probiotic viability in the product. As set by Food and Agriculture Organization (FAO) of the United Nations and the World Health Organization (WHO), the standard in order to be considered a health food with probitic addition, the product should contain per gram at least 10^6-10^7 cfu of viable probiotic bacteria. It is necessary that the bacterial cells remain stable and healthy in the manufactured product, are sufficiently viable while moving through the upper digestive tract and are able to provide positive effects upon reaching the intestine of the host.

Cell microencapsulation technology has successfully been applied in the food industry for the encapsulation of live probiotic bacteria cells to increase viability of the bacteria during processing of dairy products and for targeted delivery to the gastrointestinal tract.

Apart from dairy products, microencapsulated probiotics have also been used in non-dairy products, such as TheresweetTM which is a sweetener. It can be used as a convenient vehicle for delivery of encapsulated *Lactobacillus* to the intestine although it is not itself a dairy product.

Therapeutic Applications

Diabetes

The potential of using bioartificial pancreas, for treatment of diabetes mellitus, based on encapsulating islet cells within a semi permeable membrane is extensively being studied by scientists. These devices could eliminate the need for of immunosuppressive drugs in addition to finally solving the problem of shortage of organ donors. The use of microencapsulation would protect the islet cells from immune rejection as well as allow the use of animal cells or genetically modified insulin-producing cells. It is hoped that development of these islet encapsulated microcapsules could prevent the need for the insulin injections needed several times a day by type 1 diabetic patients. The Edmonton protocol involves implantation of human islets extracted from cadaveric donors and has shown improvements towards the treatment of type 1 diabetics who are prone to hypoglycemic unawareness. However, the two major hurdles faced in this technique are the limited availability of donor organs and with the need for immunosuppresents to prevent an immune response in the patient's body.

Several studies have been dedicated towards the development of bioartificial pancreas involving the immobilization of islets of Langerhans inside polymeric capsules. The first attempt towards this aim was demonstrated in 1980 by Lim et al. where xenograft islet cells were encapsulated inside alginate polylysine microcapsules and showed significant in vivo results for several weeks. It is envisaged that the implantation of these encapsulated cells would help to overcome the use of immunosuppressive drugs and also allow the use of xenograft cells thus obviating the problem of donor shortage.

The polymers used for islet microencapsulation are alginate, chitosan, polyethylene glycol (PEG), agarose, sodium cellulose sulfate and water-insoluble polyacrylates with alginate and PEG being commonly used polymers. With successful in vitro studies being performed using this technique, significant work in clinical trials using microencapsulated human islets is being carried out. In 2003, the use of alginate/PLO microcapsules containing islet cells for pilot phase-1 clinical trials was permitted to be carried out at the University of Perugia by the Italian Ministry of Health. In another study, the potential of clinical application of PEGylation and low doses of the immunosuppressant cyclosporine A were evaluated. The trial which began in 2005 by Novocell, now forms the phase I/II of clinical trials involving implantation of islet allografts into the subcutaneous site. However, there have been controversial studies involving human clinical trials where Living Cell technologies Ltd demonstrated the survival of functional xenogeneic cells transplanted without immunosuppressive medication for 9.5 years. However, the trial received harsh criticism from the International Xenotransplantation Association as being risky and premature. However, even though clinical trials are under way, several major issues such as biocompatibility and immuno protection need to be overcome.

Potential alternatives to encapsulating isolated islets (of either allo- or xenogeneic origin) are also being explored. Using sodium cellulose sulphate technology from Austrianova Singapore an islet cell line was encapsulated and it was demonstrated that the cells remain viable and release insulin in response to glucose. In pre-clinical studies, implanted, encapsulated cells were able to restore blood glucose levels in diabetic rats over a period of 6 months.

Cancer

The use of cell encapsulated microcapsules towards the treatment of several forms of cancer has shown great potential. One approach undertaken by researchers is through the implantation of microcapsules containing genetically modified cytokine secreting cells. An example of this was demonstrated by Cirone et al. when genetically modified IL-2 cytokine secreting non-autologous mouse myoblasts implanted into mice showed a delay in the tumor growth with an increased rate of survival of the animals. However, the efficiency of this treatment was brief due to an immune response towards the implanted microcapsules. Another approach to cancer suppression is through the use of angiogenesis inhibitors to prevent the release of growth factors which lead to the spread of tumors. The effect of implanting microcapsules loaded with xenogenic cells genetically modified to secrete endostatin, an antiangiogenic drug which causes apoptosis in tumor cells, has been extensively studied. However, this method of local delivery of microcapsules was not feasible in the treatment of patients with many tumors or in metastasis cases and has led to recent studies involving systemic implantation of the capsules.

In 1998, a murine model of pancreatic cancer was used to study the effect of implanting genetically modified cytochrome P450 expressing feline epithelial cells encapsulated in cellulose sulfate polymers for the treatment of solid tumors. The approach demonstrated for the first time the application of enzyme expressing cells to activate chemotherapeutic agents. On the basis of these results, an encapsulated cell therapy product, NovaCaps, was tested in a phaseI/II clinical trial for the treatment of pancreatic cancer in patients and has recently been designated by the European medicines agency (EMEA) as an orphan drug in Europe. A further phase I/II clinical trial using the same product confirmed the results of the first trial, demonstrating an approximate doubling of survival time in patients with stage IV pancreatic cancer. In all of these trials using cellulose sulphate, in addition to the clear anti-tumour effects, the capsules were well tolerated and there were no adverse reactions seen such as immune response to the capsules, demonstrating the biocompatible nature of the cellulose sulphate capsules. In one patient the capsules were in place for almost 2 years with no side effects.

These studies show the promising potential application of cell microcapsules towards the treatment of cancers. However, solutions to issues such as immune response leading to inflammation of the surrounding tissue at the site of capsule implantation have to be researched in detail before more clinical trials are possible.

Heart Diseases

Numerous studies have been dedicated towards the development of effective methods to enable cardiac tissue regeneration in patients after ischemic heart disease. An emerging approach to answer the problems related to ischemic tissue repair is through the use of stem cell-based therapy. However, the actual mechanism due to which this stem cell-based therapy has generative effects on cardiac function is still under investigation. Even though numerous methods have been studied for cell administration, the efficiency of the number of cells retained in the beating heart after implantation is still very low. A promising approach to overcome this problem is through the use of cell microencapsulation therapy which has shown to enable higher cell retention as compared to the injection of free stem cells into the heart.

Another strategy to improve the impact of cell based encapsulation technique towards cardiac regenerative applications is through the use of genetically modified stem cells capable of secreting angiogenic factors such as vascular endothelial growth factor (VEGF) which stimulate neovascularization and restore perfusion in the damaged ischemic heart. An example of this is shown in the study by Zang et al. where genetically modified xenogeneic CHO cells expressing VEGF were encapsulated in alginate-polylysine-alginate microcapsules and implanted into rat myocardium. It was observed that the encapsulation protected the cells from an immunorespone for three weeks and also led to an improvement in the cardiac tissue post-infarction due to increased angiogenesis.

Monoclonal Antibody Therapy

The use of monoclonal antibodies for therapy is now widespread for treatment of cancers and inflammatory diseases. Using cellulose sulphate technology, scientists have successfully encapsulated antibody producing hybridoma cells and demonstrated subsequent release of the therapeutic antibody from the capsules. The capsules containing the hybridoma cells were used in pre-clinical studies to deliver neutralising antibodies to the mouse retrovirus FrCasE, successfully preventing disease.

Other Conditions

Many other medical conditions have been targeted with encapsulation therapies, especially those involving a deficiency in some biologically derived protein. One of the most successful approaches is an external device that acts similarly to a dialysis machine, only with a reservoir of pig hepatocytes surrounding the semipermeable portion of the blood-infused tubing. This apparatus can remove toxins from the blood of patients suffering severe liver failure. Other applications that are still in development include cells that produce Ciliary-derived neurotrophic factor for the treatment of ALS and Huntington's Disease, Glial-derived neurotrophic factor for Parkinson's Disease, Erythropoietin for Anemia, and HGH for Dwarfism. In addition, monogeneic diseases such as haemophilia, Gaucher's disease and some Mucopolysaccharide disorders could also potentially be targeted by encapsulated cells expressing the protein that is otherwise lacking in the patient.

Bioactive Glass

Bioactive glasses are novel dental materials that are different from conventional glasses and are used in dentistry. Bioactive glasses are composed of calcium and phosphate, which are present in a proportion that is similar to the bone hydroxyapatite. These glasses bond to the tissue and are biocompatible.

Properties of Bioactive Glass

BAGs, as opposed to most technical glasses, are characterized by the materials' reactivity in water and in aqueous liquids. The bioactivity of BAGs is derived from their reactions with tissue fluids, resulting in the formation of a hydroxycarbonate apatite (HCA) layer on the glass.

When BAGs are brought into contact with body fluids a rapid leach of Na^+ and congruent dissolution of Ca^{2+}, PO_4^{3-} and Si^{4+} takes place at the glass surface. A polycondensated silica-rich (Si-gel) layer is formed on the glass bulk, which then serves as a template for the formation of a calcium phosphate (Ca/P) layer at its outer surface. Eventually, the Ca/P crystallizes into HCA, the composition of which corresponds to that of bone. Because of this phenomenon and their good biocompatibility, BAGs were introduced in dentistry: As substitutes for reconstruction of voids and defects of facial bones," in rehabilitation of the dentoalveolar complex, including BAG implants and regeneration of periodontal bone support."

Recently, evidence has emerged suggesting that certain compositions of BAGs create an osteoconductive response; aid in the differentiation of osteoprogenitor cells to osteoblasts and enhance bone proliferation. The essential chemical property of BAGs to release Si^+, Ca^{2+} and PO_4^{3-} in the tissue fluid, resulting in the initiation of apatite formation on the glass surface has led us to believe that it might also be quite possible to use the materials as vehicles for ectopic mineralization of the surrounding tissue. In this case, the BAGs may have therapeutic value as mineralizing agents in caries prophylactics, and also as a desensitizing agent in clinical situations where opened dentinal tubules lead to hypersensitive teeth.

Furthermore, in implantology, a coating of technically adequate BAG on the fixture surface may serve as a means to attach mucosal or dermal soft tissues to the osseointegrated construction by an HCA bridge. In addition, BAGs may also have an application in root canal therapy providing a biological seal in the form of mineral deposition inducing materials in the root canal and at the apex.

The BAGs can be employed to repair and to rebuild damaged tissues, particularly hard tissues. One point that differentiates them from other bioactive ceramics or glass-ceramic is the possibility to tailor a great chemical range of properties and of linking speed to the tissues. Therefore, it is possible to design glasses with tailored property for a specific clinical application.

The BAGs can be produced with the conventional technologies of the glass industry, but it is necessary to verify the purity of the raw materials, to avoid the contamination of impurity and the loss of volatile elements, like Na_2O, or P_2O_5. The different phases of production, so like the choice of the raw materials, influence the final features of the piece. The BAGs are soft glasses and, therefore, the final shape can be easily given with conventional tools.

The base components are usually SiO_2, Na_2O, CaO, and P_2O_5 and given below are percentages in weight of the most common BAGs.

Bioglass composition in wt%

- SiO_2-45 wt%

- Na_2O - 24.5 wt%

- CaO - 24.5 wt%

- P_2O_5-6

The abbreviation indicates that it contains 45% in weight of $SiO2$(oxide creator) and the molar rate between Ca/P is of 5:1. Glasses with significantly lower molar rate (in the form of CaO and P_2O_5) do not generate connections with the bone.

Mechanism of Bioactivity

Stage 1: It is the loss of sodium ions (Na^+) from the surface of the glass via ion exchange with hydrogen (H^+ or H_3O^+). This reaction occurs very rapidly, within minutes of material exposure to bodily fluids, and creates a de-alkalinization of the surface layer with a net negative surface charge. This stage is usually controlled by diffusion and exhibits a $t^{-1/2}$ dependence.

Stage 2: Loss of soluble silica in the form of $Si(OH)_4$ to the solution resulting from the breaking of Si-O-Si bonds and formation of Si-OH (silanols) at the glass solution interface.

This stage is usually controlled by interfacial reaction and exhibits a $t^{1.0}$ dependence. Hench has proposed that the loss of soluble silica from the surface of BAGs might be at least partially responsible for stimulating the proliferation of bone-forming cells in the area of the glass surface.

Stage 3: Condensation and repolymerization of a SiO_2-rich layer on the surface depleted in alkalis and alkaline earth cations.

Stage 4: Migration of Ca^{2+} and PO_4^{3-} groups to the surface through the SiO_2-rich layer forming a $CaO-P_2O_5$-rich film on top of the SiO_2-rich layer, followed by growth of the amorphous $CaO-P_2O_5$-rich film by incorporation of soluble calcium and phosphates from solution.

Stage 5: Crystallization of the amorphous $CaO-P_2O_5$ film by incorporation of OH^-, CO_3^{2-}, or F^- anions from solution to form a mixed hydroxyl, carbonate, fluorapatite layer.

The adsorption of proteins and other biologic moieties occurs concurrently with the first four reaction stages and is believed to contribute to the biological nature of the HCA layer. Because this surface is chemically and structurally nearly identical to natural bone mineral, the body's tissues are able to attach directly to it. As the reactivity continues, this surface HCA layer grows in thickness to form a bonding zone of 100–150 μm – A mechanically compliant interface that is essential for maintaining the bioactive bonding of the implant to the natural tissue. These surface reactions occur within the first 12–24 h of implantation.

Thus by the time osteogenic cells, such as osteoblasts or mesenchymal stem cells, infiltrate a bony defect–which normally takes 24–72 hours–they will encounter a bonelike surface, complete with organic components, and not a foreign material.

Stage 6: Adsorption of biological moieties in the SiO2-hydroxycabonate apatite layer.

Stage 7: Action of macrophages.

Stage 8: Attachment of stem cells.

Stage 9: Differentiation of stem cells.

Stage 10: Generation of matrix.

Stage 11: Mineralization of matrix.

It is this sequence of events, in which the BAG participates in the repair process that allows for the creation of a direct bond of the material to tissue. The body's normal healing and regeneration processes (stages 7–11) begin after these surface layers have begun to form. BAGs appear to minimize the duration of the macrophage and inflammatory responses that accompany any trauma, including surgery.

Implication of Bioactive Glass in Dentistry

BAG is used extensively in medicine and dentistry. The first Bioglass device used to treat conductive hearing loss by replacing the bones of the middle ear. The device was called the "Bioglass Ossicular Reconstruction Prosthesis," and trade named "MEP." It was a solid, cast Bioglass structure that acted to conduct sound from the tympanic membrane to the cochlea. The advantage of the MEP over other devices in use at the time was its ability to bond with soft tissue (tympanic membrane), as well as bone tissue. The second Bioglass device to be placed into the market was the Endosseous Ridge Maintenance Implant. The device was designed to support labial and lingual plates in natural tooth roots and to provide a more stable ridge for denture construction following tooth extraction. The devices were simple cones of 45S5 Bioglass that were placed into fresh tooth extraction sites. They bonded to the bone tissue and proved to be extremely stable, with much lower failure rates than other materials that had been used for that same purpose.

When the glass composition exceeds 52% by weight of SiO_2, the glass will bond to the bone but not to soft tissues. This finding provided the basis for clinical use of Bioglass in ossicular replacement and also for implants to maintain the alveolar ridge of edentulous patients.

Nanoparticles range from 1 nm to100 nm in size and consist of physiochemical property that does not exhibit in a bulk form where the materials display constant physical properties apart from their size. Nanoparticles hold large surface area to volume ratio which shows high binding capacity and have the potential to easily conjugate with biomolecules. BAG polymer nanocomposites are a relatively new class of bioactive materials that are suitable primarily for applications as orthopedic three-dimensional (3D) scaffolds or as bone filler materials that combine important mechanical properties and bioactivity with a polymer's great flexibility and capacity to deform under loads.Nanostructured bioglass-based materials have been created in the form of 3D scaffolds, as nanoparticles, or coatings which show comparable mechanical properties to those of natural bone. These have been created by various methods such as by sol-gel processing, unidirectional freezing of suspensions, solid freeform fabrication, electrospinning, polymer foam replication, microemulsion techniques, and others. These products have the potential of enhanced bioactivity because of the increased specific area which leads to faster dissolution and release of ions, and a higher protein adsorption

BAG particles ranging between 300 and 355 mm in diameter (BioGran) have shown in animal experiments to possess bone regenerative activities. For this reason, the material has also been used for repair of alveolar bone defects in humans and recently it has been used for sinus floor augmentation in humans, showing bone regenerative activity.

BAGs are silicates containing sodium, calcium, and phosphate as their main components. They bind to the bone by a surface layer of hydroxylapatite that forms through a chemical reaction with the glass. This chemical bonding of BAG and bone has been shown by several investigators. BAG is biocompatible, bone-bonding, and osteoconductive in humans. Good results have been achieved with this material in frontal sinus surgery.

Bioglass is not only bioactive, but it is also bacteriostatic, which may be one reason why there were no acute or late infections after frontal sinus obliteration or orbital floor reconstruction. BAG is considered to be a breakthrough in re-mineralization technology. This is because the current standard treatment for tooth remineralization and prevention of decay is slow acting and is dependent on adequate saliva as a source of calcium and phosphorus. When BAG is incorporated into toothpaste formulations, the ions released from the amorphous Ca/P layer are believed to contribute to the remineralization process of the tooth surface.

Recently, it has been demonstrated that fine particulate BAGs (<90 um) incorporated into an aqueous dentifrice have the ability to clinically reduce the tooth hypersensitivity through the occlusion of dentinal tubules by the formation of the carbonated hydroxyapatite layer.

BAGs of the $SiO_2-Na_2O-CaO-P_2O_5$ type have recently been suggested as topical root canal disinfectants.

Similarly to calcium hydroxide, the most frequently advocated interappointment dressing, BAGs disinfect their environment viathe continuous release of alkaline species in a wet environment. Calcium hydroxide and also BAG suspensions are best administered as slurries that can be applied by means of a counter angle handpiece and a lentulo spiral. However, in contrast to calcium hydroxide, BAGs do not weaken the dentin structure. They release calcium, phosphate, sodium, and silica, and thus change slowly into pure inert Ca/P particles.

BAGs cause Ca/P precipitation in their environment. Consequently, these materials transform from reactive local antiseptics into a bioactive hard tissue like structure over time. Investigators have demonstrated a significant antimicrobial effect against caries pathogens (Streptococcus mutans, Streptococcus sanguinis) upon exposure to BAG powders, as well as solution and extracts.

Advantages and Disadvantages of Bioactive Glass

The main advantage of the BAGs is the high superficial speed reaction that brings to rapid connections to the tissues. The greater disadvantages are the not optimal mechanical property and the meagre break resistance. The out bending-tensile rigidity of the greater part of the BAGs varied between 40 and 60 MPa, and they are not, therefore, usable for loading applications. Bioglasses are embedded in a biomaterial support to form prosthetics for hard tissues. Such prosthetics are biocompatible, show excellent mechanical properties and are useful for orthopedic and dental prosthetics.

The elastic modulus is in the order of 30–35 GPa, and it is very similar to that of the cortical bone. The low resistance does not hinder the use of the BAGs like covering, where the limiting factor is the resistance of the interface between the metal and the covering, so it does not hinder the use in low load or loaded in compression implantations, in shape of dust, or like bioactive phase in composites.

References

- J. F. Shackelford (editor)(1999) MSF bioceramics applications of ceramic and glass materials in medicine ISBN 0-87849-822-2

- Biomaterials, science-topics, science-education: nibib.nih.gov, Retrieved 11 May 2018

- Boch, Philippe, Niepce, Jean-Claude. (2010) Ceramic Materials: Processes, Properties and Applications. doi: 10.1002/9780470612415.ch12

- Salmons, B; Hauser, O.; Gunzburg, W. H.; Tabotta, W. (2007). "GMP production of an encapsulated cell therapy product: issues and considerations". BioProcessing Journal. 6(2): 37–44

- Nanocellulose-preparation-method-and-applications-319076893: researchgate.net, Retrieved 21 March 2018

- Kassinger, Ruth. Ceramics: From Magic Pots to Man-Made Bones. Brookfield, CT: Twenty-First Century Books, 2003, ISBN 978-0761325857

- Chai, Chou; Leong, Kam W (2007). "Biomaterials Approach to Expand and Direct Differentiation of Stem Cells". Molecular Therapy. 15 (3): 467–80. doi:10.1038/sj.mt.6300084. PMC 2365728. PMID 17264853

- Cell-encapsulation: novamatrix.biz, Retrieved 21 June 2018

- Dave RI, Shah NP (January 1997). "Viability of yoghurt and probiotic bacteria in yoghurts made from commercial starter cultures". International Dairy Journal. 7 (1): 31–41. doi:10.1016/S0958-6946(96)00046-5

Devices and Imaging

Various devices and imaging techniques are integral to the field of biomedical engineering. A medical device is used for diagnosing a health condition and for the treatment and prevention of diseases. Medical imaging is a major area in medical devices. A detailed analysis of biomedical engineering devices and imaging techniques has been provided in this chapter, such as implant, prosthesis, tomography, image registration, radiology, radiomics, etc.

Medical Device

'Medical device' means any instrument, apparatus, implement, machine, appliance, implant, reagent for in vitro use, software, material or other similar or related article, intended by the manufacturer to be used, alone or in combination, for human beings, for one or more of the specific medical purpose(s) of:

- Diagnosis, prevention, monitoring, treatment or alleviation of disease,
- Diagnosis, monitoring, treatment, alleviation of or compensation for an injury,
- Investigation, replacement, modification, or support of the anatomy or of a physiological process,
- Supporting or sustaining life,
- Control of conception,
- Disinfection of medical devices,
- Providing information by means of in vitro examination of specimens derived from the human body;

And does not achieve its primary intended action by pharmacological, immunological or metabolic means, in or on the human body, but which may be assisted in its intended function by such means.

Note: Products which may be considered to be medical devices in some jurisdictions but not in others include:

- Disinfection substances,

- Aids for persons with disabilities,

- Devices incorporating animal and/or human tissues,

- Devices for in-vitro fertilization or assisted reproduction technologies.

Active Medical Device

Any medical device the operation of which depends on a source of electrical energy or any source of power other than that directly generated by the human body or gravity and which acts by converting this energy.

Medical device relying for its functioning on a source of electrical energy or any source of power other than that directly generated by the human body or gravity. E.g.: Ultrasound scanner, lungs ventilator, X-ray machines, pacemaker, phototherapy etc.

Non-active Medical Device

Medical devices, without an integral power source. E.g.: cardiovascular stents, cardiac valves, surgical equipment, injection, infusion, dialysis etc.

Active Implantable Medical Devices

Active medical device which is intended to be totally or partially introduced, surgically or medically, into the human body or by medical intervention into a natural orifice, and which is intended to remain after the procedure.

In Vitro Diagnostic Medical Device (IVE or IVDMD)

Means any medical device which is a reagent, reagent product, calibrator, control material, kit, instrument, apparatus, equipment, or system, whether used alone or in combination, intended by the manufacturer to be used in vitro for the examination of specimens, including blood and tissue donations, derived from the human body, solely or principally for the purpose of providing information:

- Concerning a physiological or pathological state, or

- Concerning a congenital abnormality, or

- To determine the safety and compatibility with potential recipients or

- To monitor therapeutic measures.

Specimen receptacles are considered to be in vitro diagnostic medical devices. 'Specimen receptacles' are those devices, whether vacuum-type or not, specifically intended by their manufacturers for the primary containment and preservation of specimens derived from the human body for the purpose of in vitro diagnostic examination. Products for general laboratory use are not in vitro diagnostic medical devices unless such products, in view of their characteristics, are specifically intended by their manufacturer to be used for in vitro diagnostic examination.

Implant

Medical implants are devices or tissues that are placed inside or on the surface of the body. Many implants are prosthetics, intended to replace missing body parts. Other implants deliver medication, monitor body functions, or provide support to organs and tissues. Some implants are made from skin, bone or other body tissues. Others are made from metal, plastic, ceramic or other materials. Implants can be placed permanently or they can be removed once they are no longer needed. For example, stents or hip implants are intended to be permanent. But chemotherapy ports or screws to repair broken bones can be removed when they no longer needed. The risks of medical implants include surgical risks during placement or removal, infection, and implant failure. Some people also have reactions to the materials used in implants. All surgical procedures have risks. These include bruising at the surgical site, pain, swelling and redness. When your implant is inserted or removed, you should expect these types of complications. Infections are common. Most come from skin contamination at the time of surgery. If you get an infection, you may need to have a drain inserted near the implant, take medication, or even have the implant removed. Over time, your implant could move, break, or stop working properly. If this happens, you may require additional surgery to repair or replace the implant.

Implant-to-surface Communication

In implant-to-surface communication, galvanic coupling is used to send signals from an implanted device to electrodes on the skin. This allows for easy placement and repositioning of the skin electrodes to improve the quality of signal reception. However, because the signal has to travel through the skin, which is less conductive than many of the tissues inside the body, more signal attenuation occurs.

Human Cadaver Testing

A method of galvanic communication between an implanted device and surface electrodes to monitor and transmit information about anterior cruciate ligament graft tension after surgery . Two platinum electrodes (each 0.38 mm in diameter, separated by 2.5 mm) were used to inject current into the leg of a human cadaver. Electromyography (EMG) electrodes on the surface of the leg were able to detect the transmitted signals. The signals tested were sine waves with frequencies of 2–160 kHz and currents of 1–3 mA, resulting in a minimum signal attenuation of 37 dB. The attenuation increased with smaller currents, with longer distance to the surface electrodes, and with decreased inter-electrode separation of the surface EMG electrodes. In addition, the signal attenuation was sensitive to the placement of the surface electrodes in relation to the joint line. Because standard EMG electrodes were used to receive the signal, they could be easily repositioned to improve the quality of signal reception. However, the signal attenuation remained very high (37–50 dB), making signal transmission with high signal-to-noise ratios difficult.

Anesthetized Animal Testing

The implanted transmitter was integrated in an 'x-antenna', where the electrodes were integrated in two parabola-like surfaces that altered the current flow. The insulated sections of the x-antenna caused the current to flow in larger paths around the antenna and allowed for more current to be detected at the receiver electrodes. In a saline test, signal delivery using the x-antenna was found to only require 1% of the power of a traditional electrode pair. However, the diameter of the x-antenna was 9 mm, and the transmitter was designed to be implanted on the surface of the brain in between the dura and the cortex, with the signal detected by needle electrodes in the scalp. This system would be too large to be implanted inside the brain without causing significant damage.

Implant-to-implant Communication

In implant-to-implant communication, signals are transmitted from the implanted device to receiver electrodes also implanted inside the body. The implanted receiver can then be connected to equipment outside the body using a short wire or with wireless RF telemetry. In this way, less power is needed to transmit to the implanted receiver electrodes than to electrodes on the skin. However, the implanted receiver electrodes cannot be as easily repositioned as skin-mounted receiver electrodes.

Tissue Analog Testing

A system for implant-to-implant communication was developed by Wegmueller and tested in a muscle-tissue analog. The two electrodes of the transmitter galvanically coupled an alternating-current signal into the body. The signal was then detected by two receiver electrodes. Signals with frequencies of 100–500 kHz were used in order to avoid common neural frequencies, and less than 1 μA of current was used. Two different designs for the transmitting and receiving electrodes were tested: pairs of exposed copper cylinders (10 mm in length and 4 mm in diameter) and exposed copper circles (4 mm in diameter). The electrode sites were spaced 50 mm apart for both the transmitter and receiver. The copper cylinder electrodes could transmit sinusoidal signals with a loss of approximately 32 dB over 5 cm, and the copper circle electrodes had a loss of 47 dB over 5 cm. However, the electrodes were large and significant signal loss was found with any misalignment between the transmitter and receiver electrodes. The large signal losses were caused by the four-electrode design; most of the transmitted current returned to the transmitter and did not reach the receiver.

Anesthetized Animal Testing

The system used two electrodes in contact with the tissue, one for the transmitter and one for the receiver. Both electrodes were made from 50-μm diameter platinum–iridium wire. The transmitter, an insulated complementary metal–oxide–semiconductor chip less than 1 mm³ in volume, was implanted in the rat's brain and transmitted alternating-current signals to the receiver electrode, which was also implanted in the brain. Because the transmitter's circuit ground was insulated from the tissue, the path for current returning to the transmitter had higher impedance than the path through the brain to the receiver. Thus, there was a high-efficiency transfer of the signal to the recording site. Care was taken to use a charge-balanced alternating-current signal in order to avoid charge buildup or tissue damage at the electrode. Using this setup, an encoded neural signal was faithfully transmitted through brain tissue with approximately 20 dB of signal loss. A simultaneous microelectrode recording showed no obvious disruption in activity during signal transmission in the anesthetized rat's brain. The two-electrode setup of this system allowed for high efficiency transmission of the signal, but made the system vulnerable to extra current sinks in the system. If a low impedance path to ground was present, such as contact between the body and a circuit ground or a grounded water pipe, the signal would be lost.

Surface-to-surface Communication

Galvanic coupling can also be used to communicate between devices mounted on the skin. Surface-to-surface communication allows for quick and easy positioning of electrodes, fewer constraints on the size and power demands of the transmitting devices, and avoids surgical implantation. However, because the sensors are on the skin, they may be far from the sources of the signals that are being measured and can result in weak, distorted or indirect physiological measurements compared with implanted sensors. Nevertheless, these surface-to-surface signals can be combined with signals from implanted devices to create a network of sensors across and inside the body.

Human Testing

Because of the convenience and noninvasiveness of surface-to-surface systems, they can easily be tested in humans. Many laboratories have successfully used galvanic intrabody communication to transmit data between electrodes attached to the skin.

Applications

Implants can roughly be categorized into groups by application.

Sensory and Neurological

Sensory and neurological implants are used for disorders affecting the major senses and the brain, as well as other neurological disorders. They are predominately used in the treatment of conditions such as cataract, glaucoma, keratoconus, and other visual impairments; otosclerosis and other hearing loss issues, as well as middle ear diseases such as otitis media; and neurological diseases such as epilepsy, Parkinson's disease, and treatment-resistant depression. Examples include the intraocular lens, intrastromal corneal ring segment, cochlear implant, tympanostomy tube, and neurostimulator.

Cardiovascular

Cardiovascular medical devices are implanted in cases where the heart, its valves, and the rest of the circulatory system is in disorder. They are used to treat conditions such as heart failure, cardiac arrhythmia, ventricular tachycardia, valvular heart disease, angina pectoris, and atherosclerosis. Examples include the artificial heart, artificial heart valve, implantable cardioverter-defibrillator, cardiac pacemaker, and coronary stent.

Orthopedic

Orthopaedic implants help alleviate issues with the bones and joints of the body. They're used to treat bone fractures, osteoarthritis, scoliosis, spinal stenosis, and chronic pain. Examples include a wide variety of pins, rods, screws, and plates used to anchor fractured bones while they heal.

Metallic glasses based on magnesium with zinc and calcium addition are tested as the potential metallic biomaterials for biodegradable medical implants.

Patient with orthopaedic implants sometimes need to be put under magnetic resonance imaging (MRI) machine for detailed musculoskeletal study. Therefore, concerns have been raised regarding the loosening and migration of implant, heating of the implant metal which could cause thermal damage to surrounding tissues, and distortion of the MRI scan that affects the imaging results. A study of orthopaedic implants in 2005 has shown that majority of the orthopaedic implants does not react with magnetic fields under the 1.0 Tesla MRI scanning machine with the exception of external fixator clamps. However, at 7.0 Tesla, several orthopaedic implants would show significant interaction with the MRI magnetic fields, such as heel and fibular implant.

Contraception

Contraceptive implants are primarily used to prevent unintended pregnancy and treat conditions such as non-pathological forms of menorrhagia. Examples include copper- and hormone-based intrauterine devices.

Cosmetic

Cosmetic implants — often prosthetics — attempt to bring some portion of the body back to an acceptable aesthetic norm. They are used as a follow-up to mastectomy due to breast cancer, for correcting some forms of disfigurement, and modifying aspects of the body (as in buttock augmentation and chin augmentation). Examples include the breast implant, nose prosthesis, ocular prosthesis, and injectable filler.

Other Organs and Systems

Other types of organ dysfunction can occur in the systems of the body, including the gastrointestinal, respiratory, and urological systems. Implants are used in those and other locations to treat conditions such as gastroesophageal reflux disease, gastroparesis, respiratory failure, sleep apnea, urinary and fecal incontinence, and erectile dysfunction. Examples include the LINX, implantable gastric stimulator, diaphragmatic/phrenic nerve stimulator, neurostimulator, surgical mesh, and penile prosthesis.

Complications

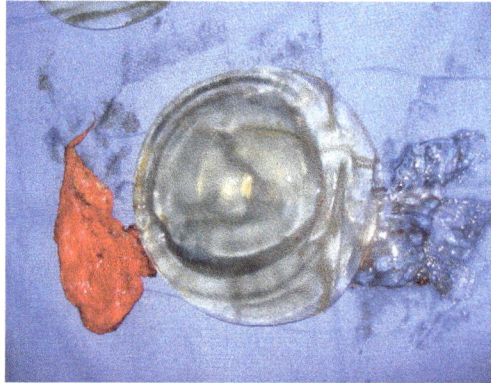

Figure: Complications can arise from implant failure.
Internal rupturing of a breast implant can lead to bacterial infection, for example.

Under ideal conditions, implants should initiate the desired host response. Ideally, the implant should not cause any undesired reaction from neighboring or distant tissues. However, the interaction between the implant and the tissue surrounding the implant can lead to complications. The process of implantation of medical devices is subjected to the same complications that other invasive medical procedures can have during or after surgery. Common complications include infection, inflammation, and pain. Other complications that can occur include risk of rejection from implant-induced coagulation and allergic foreign body response. Depending on the type of implant, the complications may vary.

When the site of an implant becomes infected during or after surgery, the surrounding tissue becomes infected by microorganisms. Three main categories of infection can occur after operation. Superficial immediate infections are caused by organisms that commonly grow near or on skin. The infection usually occurs at the surgical opening. Deep immediate infection, the second type, occurs immediately after surgery at the site of the implant. Skin-dwelling and airborne bacteria cause deep immediate infection. These bacteria enter the body by attaching to the implant's surface prior to implantation. Though not common, deep immediate infections can also occur from dormant bacteria from previous infections of the tissue at the implantation site that have been activated from being disturbed during the surgery. The last type, late infection, occurs months to years after the implantation of the implant. Late infections are caused by dormant blood-borne bacteria attached to the implant prior to implantation. The blood-borne bacteria colonize on the implant and eventually get released from it. Depending on the type of material used to make the implant, it may be infused with antibiotics to lower the risk of infections during surgery. However, only certain types of materials can be infused with antibiotics, the use of antibiotic-infused implants runs the risk of rejection by the patient since the patient may develop sensitivity to the antibiotic, and the antibiotic may not work on the bacteria.

Inflammation, a common occurrence after any surgical procedure, is the body's response to tissue damage as a result of trauma, infection, intrusion of foreign materials, or local cell death, or as a part of an immune response. Inflammation starts with the rapid dilation of local capillaries to supply the local tissue with blood. The inflow of blood causes the tissue to become swollen and may cause cell death. The excess blood, or edema, can activate pain receptors at the tissue. The site of the inflammation becomes warm from local disturbances of fluid flow and the increased cellular activity to repair the tissue or remove debris from the site.

Implant-induced coagulation is similar to the coagulation process done within the body to prevent blood loss from damaged blood vessels. However, the coagulation process is triggered from proteins that become attached to the implant surface and lose their shapes. When this occurs, the protein changes conformation and different activation sites become exposed, which may trigger an immune system response where the body attempts to attack the implant to remove the foreign material. The trigger of the immune system response can be accompanied by inflammation. The immune system response may lead to chronic inflammation where the implant is rejected and has to be removed from the body. The immune system may encapsulate the implant as an attempt to remove the foreign material from the site of the tissue by encapsulating the implant in fibrinogen and platelets. The encapsulation of the implant can lead to further complications, since the thick layers of fibrous encapsulation may prevent the implant from performing the desired functions. Bacteria may attack the fibrous encapsulation and become embedded into the fibers. Since the layers of fibers are thick, antibiotics may not be able to reach the bacteria and the bacteria may grow and infect the surrounding tissue. In order to remove the bacteria, the implant would have to be removed. Lastly, the immune system may accept the presence of the implant and repair and remodel the surrounding tissue. Similar responses occur when the body initiates an allergic foreign body response. In the case of an allergic foreign body response, the implant would have to be removed.

Prosthesis

Prosthesis is an artificial substitute for a missing part of the body. The artificial parts that are most commonly thought of as prostheses are those that replace lost arms and legs, but bone, artery, and heart valve replacements are common, and artificial eyes and teeth are also correctly termed prostheses. The term is sometimes extended to cover such things as eyeglasses and hearing aids, which improve the functioning of a part. The medical specialty that deals with prostheses is called prosthetics. The origin of prosthetics as a science is attributed to the 16th-century French surgeon Ambroise Paré. Later workers developed upper-extremity replacements, including metal hands made either in one piece or with movable parts. The solid metal hand of the 16th and 17th centuries later gave way in great measure to a single hook or a leather-covered, nonfunctioning hand attached to the forearm by a leather or wooden shell. Improvement in the design of prostheses and increased acceptance of their use have accompanied major wars.

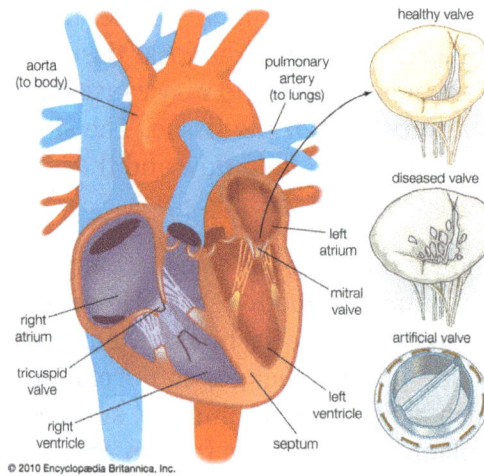

Figure: A normal heart valve compared with an artificial heart valve

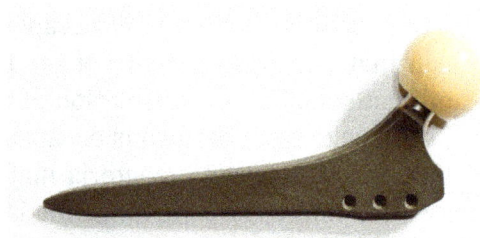

Figure: hip prosthesis. A titanium hip prosthesis.

One type of below-knee prosthesis is made from plastic and fits the below-knee stump with total contact. It is held on either by means of a strap that passes above the kneecap or by means of rigid metal knee hinges attached to a leather thigh corset. Weight bearing is accomplished by pressure of the prosthesis against the tendon that extends from the kneecap to the lower legbone. In addition, a foot piece is commonly used that consists of a solid foot and ankle with layers of rubber in the heel to give a cushioning effect.

There are two main types of above-knee prostheses:

(1) The prosthesis held on by means of a belt around the pelvis or suspended from the shoulder by straps and

(2) The prosthesis kept in contact with the leg stump by suction, the belt and shoulder straps being eliminated.

The more complicated prosthesis used in cases of amputation through the hip joint or half of the pelvis usually consists of a plastic socket, in which the person virtually sits; a mechanical hip joint of metal; and a leather, plastic, or wooden thigh piece with the mechanical knee, shin portion, and foot.

Arm prostheses came to be made of plastic, frequently reinforced with glass fibres.

The below-elbow prosthesis consists of a single plastic shell and a metal wrist joint to which is attached a terminal device, either a hook or a hand. The person wears a shoulder harness made of webbing, from which a steel cable extends to the terminal device. When the person shrugs the shoulder, thus tightening the cable, the terminal device opens and closes. In certain cases the biceps muscle may be attached to the prosthesis by a surgical operation known as cineplasty. This procedure makes it possible to dispense with the shoulder harness and allows finer control of the terminal device. The above-elbow prosthesis has, in addition to the forearm shell, an upper-arm plastic shell and a mechanical, locking elbow joint. This complicates its use, inasmuch as there must be one cable control for the terminal device and another control to lock and unlock the elbow. The most complicated upper-extremity prosthesis, which used in cases of amputation through the shoulder, includes a plastic shoulder cap extending over the chest and back. Usually no shoulder rotation is possible, but the mechanical elbow and terminal device function as in other arm prostheses.

A metal hook that opens and closes as two fingers is the most commonly used terminal device and the most efficient. This is a metal mechanical hand covered by a rubber glove of a colour similar to that of the patient's remaining hand. Many attempts have been made to use electrical energy as the source of hook or hand control. This is done primarily by building into the arm prosthesis electrodes that are activated by the patient's own muscle contractions. The electric current generated by these muscle contractions is then amplified by means of electrical components and batteries to control the terminal device. Such an arrangement is referred to as a myoelectrical control system.

Breast prostheses are used after mastectomy. External prostheses may be worn, but surgical reconstruction of the breast, involving implantation of prosthesis, became increasingly common from the 1970s.

Types

A person's prosthesis should be designed and assembled according to the person's appearance and functional needs. For instance, a person may need a transradial prosthesis, but need to choose between an aesthetic functional device, a myoelectric device, a body-powered device, or an activity specific device. The person's future goals and economical capabilities may help them choose between one or more devices.

Craniofacial prostheses include intra-oral and extra-oral prostheses. Extra-oral prostheses are further divided into hemifacial, auricular (ear), nasal, orbital and ocular. Intra-oral prostheses include dental prostheses such as dentures, obturators, and dental implants.

Prostheses of the neck include larynx substitutes, trachea and upper esophageal replacements.

Somato prostheses of the torso include breast prostheses which may be either single or bilateral, full breast devices or nipple prostheses.

Penile prostheses are used to treat erectile dysfunction.

Limb Prostheses

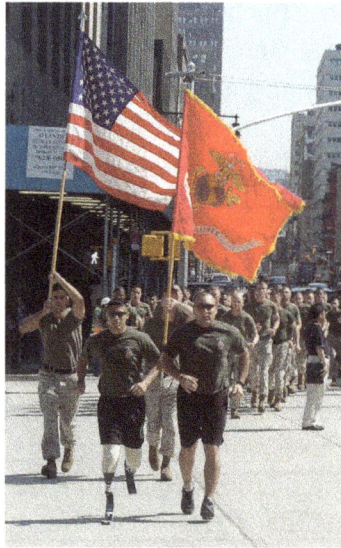

Figure: A United States Marine with bilateral prosthetic legs leads a formation run

Limb prostheses include both upper- and lower-extremity prostheses.

Upper-extremity prostheses are used at varying levels of amputation: forequarter, shoulder disarticulation, transhumeral prosthesis, elbow disarticulation, transradial prosthesis, wrist disarticulation, full hand, partial hand, finger, partial finger. A transradial prosthesis is an artificial limb that replaces an arm missing below the elbow.

Upper limb prostheses can be categorized in three main categories: Passive devices, Body Powered devices, Externally Powered (myoelectric) devices. Passive devices can either be passive hands, mainly used for cosmetic purpose, or passive tools, mainly used for specific activities (e.g. leisure or vocational). An extensive overview and classification of passive devices can be found in a literature review by Maat *et.al*. A passive device can be static, meaning the device has no movable parts, or it can be adjustable, meaning its configuration can be adjusted (e.g. adjustable hand opening). Despite the absence of active grasping, passive devices are very useful in bimanual tasks that require fixation or support of an object, or for gesticulation in social interaction. According to scientific data a third of the upper limb amputees worldwide use a passive prosthetic hand. Body Powered or cable operated limbs work by attaching a harness and cable around the opposite shoulder of the damaged arm. The third category of prosthetic devices available is myoelectric arms. These work by sensing, via electrodes, when the muscles in the upper arm move, causing an artificial hand to open or close. In the prosthetics industry, a trans-radial prosthetic arm is often referred to as a "BE" or below elbow prosthesis.

Lower-extremity prostheses provide replacements at varying levels of amputation. These include hip disarticulation, transfemoral prosthesis, knee disarticulation, transtibial prosthesis, Syme's amputation, foot, partial foot, and toe. The two main sub-categories of lower extremity prosthetic devices are trans-tibial (any amputation transecting the tibia bone or a congenital anomaly resulting in a tibial deficiency) and trans-femoral.

A transfemoral prosthesis is an artificial limb that replaces a leg missing above the knee. Transfemoral amputees can have a very difficult time regaining normal movement. In general, a transfemoral amputee must use approximately 80% more energy to walk than a person with two whole legs. This is due to the complexities in movement associated with the knee. In newer and more improved designs, hydraulics, carbon fiber, mechanical linkages, motors, computer microprocessors, and innovative combinations of these technologies are employed to give more control to the user. In the prosthetics industry a trans-femoral prosthetic leg is often referred to as an "AK" or above the knee prosthesis.

A transtibial prosthesis is an artificial limb that replaces a leg missing below the knee. A transtibial amputee is usually able to regain normal movement more readily than someone with a transfemoral amputation, due in large part to retaining the knee, which allows for easier movement. Lower extremity prosthetics describes artificially replaced limbs located at the hip level or lower. In the prosthetics industry a trans-tibial prosthetic leg is often referred to as a "BK" or below the knee prosthesis.

Physical therapists are trained to teach a person to walk with a leg prosthesis. To do so, the physical therapist may provide verbal instructions and may also help guide the person using touch, or tactile cues. This may be done in a clinic or home. There is some research suggesting that such training in the home may be more successful if the treatment includes the use of a treadmill. Using a treadmill, along with the physical therapy treatment, helps the person to experience many of the challenges of walking with a prosthesis.

In the United Kingdom, 75% of lower limb amputations are performed due to inadequate circulation (dysvascularity). This condition is often associated with many other medical conditions (co-morbidities) including diabetes and heart disease that may make it a challenge to recover and use a prosthetic limb to regain mobility and independence. For people who have inadequate circulation and have lost a lower limb, there is insufficient evidence due to a lack of research, to inform them regarding their choice of prosthetic rehabilitation approaches.

Lower extremity prostheses are often categorized by the level of amputation or after the name of a surgeon:

- Transfemoral (Above-knee)

- Transtibial (Below-knee)

- Ankle disarticulation (e.g.: Syme amputation)

- Knee disarticulation

- Hemi-pelvictomy (Hip disarticulation)

- Partial foot amputations (Pirogoff, Talo-Navicular and Calcaneo-cuboid (Chopart), Tarso-metatarsal (Lisfranc), Trans-metatarsal, Metatarsal-phalangeal, Ray amputations, toe amputations).

- Van Nes rotationplasty

Prosthetic Raw Materials

Prosthetic are made lightweight for better convenience for the amputee. Some of these materials include:

- Plastics:
  - Polyethylene
  - Polypropylene
  - Acrylics
  - Polyurethane
- Wood (early prosthetics)
- Rubber (early prosthetics)
- Lightweight metals:

- ○ Titanium
- ○ Aluminum
- Composites:
  - ○ Carbon fibre

Wheeled prostheses have also been used extensively in the rehabilitation of injured domestic animals, including dogs, cats, pigs, rabbits, and turtles.

Body-powered Arms

Current technology allows body powered arms to weigh around one-half to one-third of what a myoelectric arm does.

Sockets

Current body-powered arms contain sockets that are built from hard epoxy or carbon fiber. These sockets or "interfaces" can be made more comfortable by lining them with a softer, compressible foam material that provides padding for the bone prominences. A self-suspending or supra-condylar socket design is useful for those with short to mid-range below elbow absence. Longer limbs may require the use of a locking roll-on type inner liner or more complex harnessing to help augment suspension.

Wrists

Wrist units are either screw-on connectors featuring the UNF 1/2-20 thread (USA) or quick-release connector, of which there are different models.

Voluntary Opening and Voluntary Closing

Two types of body-powered systems exist, voluntary opening "pull to open" and voluntary closing "pulls to close". Virtually all "split hook" prostheses operate with a voluntary opening type system.

More modern "prehensors" called GRIPS utilize voluntary closing systems. The differences are significant. Users of voluntary opening systems rely on elastic bands or springs for gripping force, while users of voluntary closing systems rely on their own body power and energy to create gripping force.

Voluntary closing users can generate prehension forces equivalent to the normal hand, upwards to or exceeding one hundred pounds. Voluntary closing GRIPS require constant tension to grip, like a human hand, and in that property, they do come closer to matching human hand performance. Voluntary opening split hook users are limited to forces their rubber or springs can generate which usually is below 20 pounds.

Feedback

An additional difference exists in the biofeedback created that allows the user to "feel" what is being held. Voluntary opening systems once engaged provide the holding force so that they operate like a passive vice at the end of the arm. No gripping feedback is provided once the hook has closed around the object being held. Voluntary closing systems provide directly proportional control and biofeedback so that the user can feel how much force that they are applying.

A recent study showed that by stimulating the median and ulnar nerves, according to the information provided by the artificial sensors from a hand prosthesis, physiologically appropriate (near-natural) sensory information could be provided to an amputee. This feedback enabled the participant to effectively modulate the grasping force of the prosthesis with no visual or auditory feedback.

Researchers from École Polytechnique Fédérale De Lausanne in Switzerland and the Scuola Superiore Sant'Anna in Italy, implanted the electrodes into the amputee's arm in February 2013. The study, published Wednesday in *Science Translational Medicine*, details the first time sensory feedback has been restored allowing an amputee to control an artificial limb in real-time. With wires linked to nerves in his upper arm, the Danish patient was able to handle objects and instantly receive a sense of touch through the special artificial hand that was created by Silvestro Micera and researchers both in Switzerland and Italy.

Terminal Devices

Terminal devices contain a range of hooks, prehensors, hands or other devices.

Hooks

Voluntary opening split hook systems are simple, convenient, light, robust, versatile and relatively affordable.

A hook does not match a normal human hand for appearance or overall versatility, but its material tolerances can exceed and surpass the normal human hand for mechanical stress (one can even use a hook to slice open boxes or as a hammer whereas the same is not possible with a normal hand), for thermal stability (one can use a hook to grip items from boiling water, to turn meat on a grill, to hold a match until it has burned down completely) and for chemical hazards (as a metal hook withstands acids or lye, and does not react to solvents like a prosthetic glove or human skin).

Hands

Prosthetic hands are available in both voluntary opening and voluntary closing versions and because of their more complex mechanics and cosmetic glove covering require a relatively large activation force, which, depending on the type of harness used, may be uncomfortable. A recent study by the Delft University of Technology, The Netherlands, showed that the development of mechanical prosthetic hands has been neglected during the past decades. The study showed that the pinch force level of most current mechanical hands is too low for practical use. The best tested hand was a prosthetic hand developed around 1945. In 2017 however, a research has been started with bionic hands by Laura Hruby of the Medical University of Vienna. Some companies are also producing robotic hands with integrated forearm, for fitting unto a patient's upper arm.

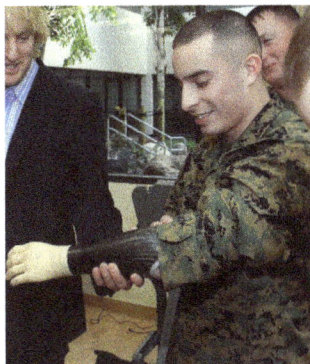

Actor Owen Wilson gripping the myoelectric prosthetic arm of a United States Marine

Commercial Providers and Materials

Hosmer and Otto Bock are major commercial hook providers. Mechanical hands are sold by Hosmer and Otto Bock as well; the Becker Hand is still manufactured by the Becker family. Prosthetic hands may be fitted with standard stock or custom-made cosmetic looking silicone gloves. But regular work gloves may be worn as well. Other terminal devices include the V2P Prehensor, a versatile robust gripper that allows customers to modify aspects of it, Texas Assist Devices (with a whole assortment of tools) and TRS that offers a range of terminal devices for sports. Cable harnesses can be built using aircraft steel cables, ball hinges, and self-lubricating cable sheaths. Some prosthetics have been designed specifically for use in salt water.

Lower-extremity Prosthetics

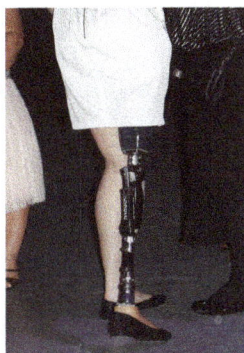

A prosthetic leg worn by Ellie Cole

Lower-extremity prosthetics describes artificially replaced limbs located at the hip level or lower. Concerning all ages Ephraim found a worldwide estimate of all-cause lower-extremity amputations of 2.0–5.9 per 10,000 inhabitants. For birth prevalence rates of congenital limb deficiency they found an estimate between 3.5–7.1 cases per 10,000 births.

The two main subcategories of lower extremity prosthetic devices are trans-tibial (any amputation transecting the tibia bone or a congenital anomaly resulting in a tibial deficiency), and trans-femoral (any amputation transecting the femur bone or a congenital anomaly resulting in a femoral deficiency). In the prosthetic industry, a trans-tibial prosthetic leg is often referred to as a "BK" or below the knee prosthesis while the trans-femoral prosthetic leg is often referred to as an "AK" or above the knee prosthesis.

Other, less prevalent lower extremity cases include the following:

1. Hip disarticulations – This usually refers to when an amputee or congenitally challenged patient has either an amputation or anomaly at or in close proximity to the hip joint.

2. Knee disarticulations – This usually refers to an amputation through the knee disarticulating the femur from the tibia.

3. Symes – This is an ankle disarticulation while preserving the heel pad.

Socket

The socket serves as an interface between the residuum and the prosthesis, ideally allowing comfortable weight-bearing, movement control and proprioception. Socket issues, such as discomfort and skin breakdown, are rated among the most important issues faced by lower-limb amputees.

Shank and Connectors

This part creates distance and support between the knee-joint and the foot (in case of an upper-leg prosthesis) or between the socket and the foot. The type of connectors that are used between the shank and the knee/foot determines whether the prosthesis is modular or not. Modular means that the angle and the displacement of the foot in respect to the socket can be changed after fitting. In developing countries prosthesis mostly are non-modular, in order to reduce cost. When considering children modularity of angle and height is important because of their average growth of 1.9 cm annually.

Foot

Providing contact to the ground, the foot provides shock absorption and stability during stance. Additionally it influences gait biomechanics by its shape and stiffness. This is because the trajectory of the center of pressure (COP) and the angle of the ground reaction forces is determined by the shape and stiffness of the foot and needs to match the subject's build in order to produce a normal gait pattern. Andrysek (2010) found 16 different types of feet, with greatly varying results concerning durability and biomechanics. The main problem found in current feet is durability; endurance ranging from 16–32 months These results are for adults and will probably be worse for children due to higher activity levels and scale effects. Evidence comparing different types of feet and ankle prosthetic devices is not strong enough to determine if one mechanism of ankle/foot is superior to another. When deciding on a device, the cost of the device, a person's functional need, and the availability of a particular device should be considered.

Knee Joint

In case of a trans-femoral amputation, there also is a need for a complex connector providing articulation, allowing flexion during swing-phase but not during stance.

Microprocessor Control

To mimic the knee's functionality during gait, microprocessor-controlled knee joints have been developed that control the flexion of the knee. Some examples are Otto Bock's C-leg, introduced in 1997, Ossur's Rheo Knee, released in 2005, the Power Knee by Ossur, introduced in 2006, the Plié Knee from Freedom Innovations and DAW Industries' Self Learning Knee (SLK).

The idea was originally developed by Kelly James, a Canadian engineer, at the University of Alberta.

A microprocessor is used to interpret and analyze signals from knee-angle sensors and moment sensors. The microprocessor receives signals from its sensors to determine the type of motion being employed by the amputee. Most microprocessor controlled knee-joints are powered by a battery housed inside the prosthesis.

The sensory signals computed by the microprocessor are used to control the resistance generated by hydraulic cylinders in the knee-joint. Small valves control the amount of hydraulic fluid that can pass into and out of the cylinder, thus regulating the extension and compression of a piston connected to the upper section of the knee.

The main advantage of a microprocessor-controlled prosthesis is a closer approximation to an amputee's natural gait. Some allow amputees to walk near walking speed or run. Variations in speed are also possible and are taken into account by sensors and communicated to the microprocessor, which adjusts to these changes accordingly. It also enables the amputees to walk downstairs with a step-over-step approach, rather than the one step at a time approach used with mechanical knees. There is some research suggesting that people with microprocessor-controlled prostheses report greater satisfaction and improvement in functionality, residual limb health, and safety.

People may be able to perform everyday activities at greater speeds, even while multitasking, and reduce their risk of falls.

However, some have some significant drawbacks that impair its use. They can be susceptible to water damage and thus great care must be taken to ensure that the prosthesis remains dry.

Myoelectric

A myoelectric prosthesis uses the electrical tension generated every time a muscle contracts, as information. This tension can be captured from voluntarily contracted muscles by electrodes applied on the skin to control the movements of the prosthesis, such as elbow flexion/extension, wrist supination/pronation (rotation) or opening/closing of the fingers. Prosthesis of this type utilizes the residual neuromuscular system of the human body to control the functions of an electric powered prosthetic hand, wrist, elbow or foot. This is different from an electric switch prosthesis, which requires straps and/or cables actuated by body movements to actuate or operate switches that control the movements of the prosthesis. There is no clear evidence concluding that myoelectric upper extremity prostheses function better than body-powered prostheses. Advantages to using a myoelectric upper extremity prosthesis include the potential for improvement in cosmetic appeal (this type of prosthesis may have a more natural look), may be better for light everyday activities, and may be beneficial for people experiencing phantom limb pain. When compared to a body-powered prosthesis, a myoelectric prosthesis may not be as durable, may have a longer training time, may require more adjustments, may need more maintenance, and does not provide feedback to the user.

The USSR was the first to develop a myoelectric arm in 1958, while the first myoelectric arm became commercial in 1964 by the Central Prosthetic Research Institute of the USSR, and distributed by the Hangar Limb Factory of the UK.

Researchers at the Rehabilitation Institute of Chicago announced in September 2013 that they have developed a robotic leg that translates neural impulses from the user's thigh muscles into movement, which is the first prosthetic leg to do so. It is currently in testing.

Robotic Prostheses

Robots can be used to generate objective measures of patient's impairment and therapy outcome, assist in diagnosis, customize therapies based on patient's motor abilities, and assure compliance with treatment regimens and maintain patient's records. It is shown in many studies that there is a significant improvement in upper limb motor function after stroke using robotics for upper limb rehabilitation. In order for a robotic prosthetic limb to work, it must have several components to integrate it into the body's function: Biosensors detect signals from the user's nervous or muscular systems. It then relays this information to a controller located inside the device, and processes feedback from the limb and actuator, e.g., position or force, and sends it to the controller. Examples include surface electrodes that detect electrical activity on the skin, needle electrodes implanted in muscle, or solid-state electrode arrays with nerves growing through them. One type of these biosensors is employed in myoelectric prostheses.

A device known as the controller is connected to the user's nerve and muscular systems and the device itself. It sends intention commands from the user to the actuators of the device and interprets feedback from the mechanical and biosensors to the user. The controller is also responsible for the monitoring and control of the movements of the device.

An actuator mimics the actions of a muscle in producing force and movement. Examples include a motor that aids or replaces original muscle tissue.

Targeted muscle reinnervation (TMR) is a technique in which motor nerves, which previously controlled muscles on an amputated limb, are surgically rerouted such that they reinnervate a small region of a large, intact muscle, such as the pectoralis major. As a result, when a patient thinks about moving the thumb of his missing hand, a small area of muscle on his chest will contract instead. By placing sensors over the reinnervated muscle, these contractions can be made to control the movement of an appropriate part of the robotic prosthesis.

A variant of this technique is called targeted sensory reinnervation (TSR). This procedure is similar to TMR, except that sensory nerves are surgically rerouted to skin on the chest, rather than motor nerves rerouted to muscle. Recently, robotic limbs have improved in their ability to take signals from the human brain and translate those signals into motion in the artificial limb. DARPA, the Pentagon's research division, is working to make even more advancements in this area. Their desire is to create an artificial limb that ties directly into the nervous system.

Robotic Arms

Advancements in the processors used in myoelectric arms have allowed developers to make gains in fine-tuned control of the prosthetic. The Boston Digital Arm is a recent artificial limb that has taken advantage of these more advanced processors. The arm allows movement in five axes and allows the arm to be programmed for a more customized feel. Recently the i-Limb hand, invented in Edinburgh, Scotland, by David Gow has become the first commercially available hand prosthesis with five individually powered digits. The hand also possesses a manually rotatable thumb which is operated passively by the user and allows the hand to grip in precision, power, and key grip modes.

Another neural prosthetic is Johns Hopkins University Applied Physics Laboratory Proto 1. Besides the Proto 1, the university also finished the Proto 2 in 2010. Early in 2013, Max Ortiz Catalan and Rickard Brånemark of the Chalmers University of Technology, and Sahlgrenska University Hospital in Sweden, succeeded in making the first robotic arm which is mind-controlled and can be permanently attached to the body (using osseointegration).

An approach that is very useful is called arm rotation which is common for unilateral amputees which is an amputation that affects only one side of the body; and also essential for bilateral amputees, a person who is missing or has had amputated either both arms or legs, to carry out activities of daily living. This involves inserting a small permanent magnet into the distal end of the residual bone of subjects with upper limb amputations. When a subject rotates the residual arm, the magnet will rotate with the residual bone, causing a change in magnetic field distribution. EEG (electroencephalogram) signals, detected using small flat metal discs attached to the scalp, essentially decoding human brain activity used for physical movement, is used to control the robotic limbs. This allows the user to control the part directly.

Robotic Legs

Prosthesis Design

The main goal of a robotic prosthesis is to provide active actuation during gait to improve the biomechanics of gait, including, among other things, stability, symmetry, or energy expenditure for amputees. There are several powered prosthetic legs currently on the market, including fully powered legs, in which actuators directly drive the joints, and semi-active legs, which use small amounts of energy and a small actuator to change the mechanical properties of the leg but do not inject net positive energy into gait. Specific examples include The emPOWER from BionX, the Proprio Foot from Ossur, and the Elan Foot from Endolite. Various research groups have also experimented with robotic legs over the last decade. Central issues being researched include designing the behavior of the device during stance and swing phases, recognizing the current ambulation task, and various mechanical design problems such as robustness, weight, battery-life/efficiency, and noise-level. However, scientists from Stanford University and Seoul National University has developed artificial nerves system that will help prosthetic limbs feel. This synthetic nerve system enables prosthetic limbs sense braille, feel the sense of touch and respond to the environment.

Attachment to the Body

Most prostheses can be attached to the exterior of the body, in a non-permanent way. Some others however can be attached in a permanent way. One such example is exo-prostheses.

Direct Bone Attachment and Osseointegration

Osseointegration is a method of attaching the artificial limb to the body. This method is also sometimes referred to as exoprosthesis (attaching an artificial limb to the bone), or endo-exoprosthesis.

The stump and socket method can cause significant pain in the amputee, which is why the direct bone attachment has been explored extensively. The method works by inserting a titanium bolt into the bone at the end of the stump. After several months the bone attaches itself to the titanium bolt and an abutment is attached to the titanium bolt. The abutment extends out of the stump and the (removable) artificial limb is then attached to the abutment. Some of the benefits of this method include the following:

- Better muscle control of the prosthetic.

- The ability to wear the prosthetic for an extended period of time; with the stump and socket method this is not possible.

- The ability for transfemoral amputees to drive a car.

The main disadvantage of this method is that amputees with the direct bone attachment cannot have large impacts on the limb, such as those experienced during jogging, because of the potential for the bone to break.

Cosmesis

Cosmetic prosthesis has long been used to disguise injuries and disfigurements. With advances in modern technology, cosmesis, the creation of lifelike limbs made from silicone or PVC has been made possible. Such prosthetics, including artificial hands, can now be designed to simulate the appearance of real hands, complete with freckles, veins, hair, fingerprints and even tattoos. Custom-made cosmeses are generally more expensive (costing thousands of U.S. dollars, depending on the level of detail), while standard cosmeses come premade in a variety of sizes, although they are often not as realistic as their custom-made counterparts. Another option is the custom-made silicone cover, which can be made to match a person's skin tone but not details such as freckles or wrinkles. Cosmeses are attached to the body in any number of ways, using an adhesive, suction, form-fitting, stretchable skin, or a skin sleeve.

Cognition

Unlike neuromotor prostheses, neurocognitive prostheses would sense or modulate neural function in order to physically reconstitute or augment cognitive processes such as executive function, attention, language, and memory. No neurocognitive prostheses are currently available but the development of implantable neurocognitive brain-computer interfaces has been proposed to help treat conditions such as stroke, traumatic brain injury, cerebral palsy, autism, and Alzheimer's disease. The recent field of Assistive Technology for Cognition concerns the development of technologies to augment human cognition. Scheduling devices such as Neuropage remind users with memory impairments when to perform certain activities, such as visiting the doctor. Micro-prompting devices such as PEAT, AbleLink and Guide have been used to aid users with memory and executive function problems perform activities of daily living.

Cost and Source Freedom

High-cost

In the USA a typical prosthetic limb costs anywhere between $15,000 and $90,000, depending on the type of limb desired by the patient. With medical insurance, a patient will typically pay 10%–50% of the total cost of a prosthetic limb, while the insurance company will cover the rest of the cost. The percent that the patient pays varies on the type of insurance plan, as well as the limb requested by the patient. In the United Kingdom, much of Europe, Australia and New Zealand the entire cost of prosthetic limbs is met by state funding or statutory insurance. For example, in Australia prostheses are fully funded by state schemes in the case of amputation due to disease, and by workers compensation or traffic injury insurance in the case of most traumatic amputations. The National Disability Insurance Scheme, which is being rolled out nationally between 2017 and 2020 also pays for prostheses.

Transradial (below the elbow amputation) and transtibial prostheses (below the knee amputation) typically cost between US $6,000 and $8,000, while transfemoral (above the knee amputation) and transhumeral prosthetics (above the elbow amputation) cost approximately twice as much with a range of $10,000 to $15,000 and can sometimes reach costs of $35,000. The cost of an artificial limb often recurs, while a limb typically needs to be replaced every 3–4 years due to wear and tear of everyday use. In addition, if the socket has fit issues, the socket must be replaced within several months from the onset of pain. If height is an issue, components such as pylons can be changed.

Not only does the patient need to pay for their multiple prosthetic limbs, but they also need to pay for physical and occupational therapy that come along with adapting to living with an artificial limb. Unlike the reoccurring cost of the prosthetic limbs, the patient will typically only pay the $2000 to $5000 for therapy during the first year or two of living as an amputee. Once the patient is strong and comfortable with their new limb, they will not be required to go to therapy anymore. Throughout one's life, it is projected that a typical amputee will go through $1.4 million worth of treatment, including surgeries, prosthetics, as well as therapies.

Low-cost

Low-cost above-knee prostheses often provide only basic structural support with limited function. This function is often achieved with crude, non-articulating, unstable, or manually locking knee joints. A limited number of organizations, such as the International Committee of the Red Cross (ICRC), create devices for developing countries. Their device which is manufactured by CR Equipments is a single-axis, manually operated locking polymer prosthetic knee joint.

Table: List of knee joint technologies based on the literature review.

Name of technology (country of origin)	Brief description	Highest level of evidence
ICRC knee (Switzerland)	Single-axis with manual lock	Independent field
ATLAS knee (UK)	Weight-activated friction	Independent field
POF/OTRC knee (US)	Single-axis with ext. assist	Field
DAV/Seattle knee (US)	Compliant polycentric	Field

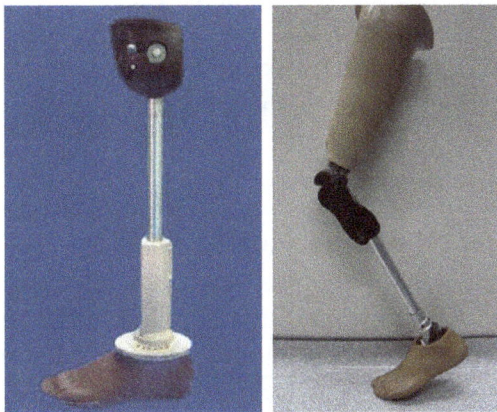

Figure: Low-cost above-knee prosthetic limbs: ICRC Knee (left) and LC Knee (right)

A plan for a low-cost artificial leg, designed by Sébastien Dubois, was featured at the 2007 International Design Exhibition and award show in Copenhagen, Denmark, where it won the Index: Award. It would be able to create an energy-return prosthetic leg for US $8.00, composed primarily of fiberglass.

Prior to the 1980s, foot prostheses merely restored basic walking capabilities. These early devices can be characterized by a simple artificial attachment connecting one's residual limb to the ground.

The introduction of the Seattle Foot (Seattle Limb Systems) in 1981 revolutionized the field, bringing the concept of an Energy Storing Prosthetic Foot to the fore. Other companies soon followed suit, and before long, there were multiple models of energy storing prostheses on the market. Each model utilized some variation of a compressible heel. The heel is compressed during initial ground contact, storing energy which is then returned during the latter phase of ground contact to help propel the body forward.

Since then, the foot prosthetics industry has been dominated by steady, small improvements in performance, comfort, and marketability.

With 3D printers, it is possible to manufacture a single product without having to have metal molds, so the costs can be drastically reduced.

Jaipur Foot, an artificial limb from Jaipur, India, costs about US$40.

Open-source Robotic Prothesis

There is currently an open-design Prosthetics forum known as the "Open Prosthetics Project". The group employs collaborators and volunteers to advance Prosthetics technology while attempting to lower the costs of these necessary devices. Open Bionics is a company that is developing open-source robotic prosthetic hands. It uses 3D printing to manufacture the devices and low-cost 3D scanners to fit them, with the aim of lowering the cost of fabricating custom prosthetics. A review study on a wide range of printed prosthetic hands, found that although 3D printing technology holds a promise for individualized prosthesis design, it is not necessarily cheaper when all costs are included. The same study also found that evidence on the functionality, durability and user acceptance of 3D printed hand prostheses is still lacking.

Low-cost Prosthetics for Children

In the USA an estimate was found of 32,500 children (<21 years) that suffer from major pediatric amputation, with 5,525 new cases each year, of which 3,315 congenital. Carr et al. (1998) investigated amputations caused by landmines for Afghanistan, Bosnia and Herzegovina, Cambodia and Mozambique among children (<14 years), showing estimates of respectively 4.7, 0.19, 1.11 and 0.67 per 1000 children. Mohan (1986) indicated in India a total of 424,000 amputees (23,500 annually), of which 10.3% had an onset of disability below the age of 14, amounting to a total of about 43,700 limb deficient children in India alone.

Few low-cost solutions have been created especially for children. Underneath some of them can be found.

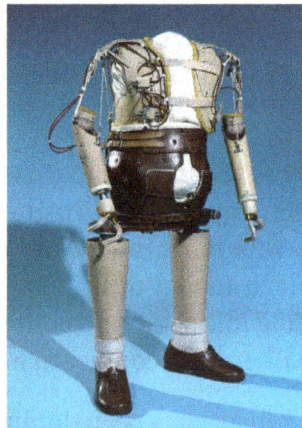

Artificial limbs for a juvenile thalidomide survivor

Pole and Crutch

This hand-held pole with leather support band or platform for the limb is one of the simplest and cheapest solutions found. It serves well as a short-term solution, but is prone to rapid contracture formation if the limb is not stretched daily through a series of range-of motion (RoM) sets.

Bamboo, PVC or Plaster Limbs

This also fairly simple solution comprises a plaster socket with a bamboo or PVC pipe at the bottom, optionally attached to a prosthetic foot. This solution prevents contractures because the knee is moved through its full RoM. The David Werner Collection, an online database for the assistance of disabled village children, displays manuals of production of these solutions.

Adjustable Bicycle Limb

This solution is built using a bicycle seat post up side down as foot, generating flexibility and (length) adjustability. It is a very cheap solution, using locally available materials.

Sathi Limb

It is an endoskeletal modular lower limb from India, which uses thermoplastic parts. Its main advantages are the small weight and adaptability.

Monolimb

Monolimbs are non-modular prostheses and thus require more experienced prosthetist for correct fitting, because alignment can barely be changed after production. However, their durability on average is better than low-cost modular solutions.

Cultural and Social Theory Perspectives

A number of theorists have explored the meaning and implications of prosthetic extension of the body. Elizabeth Grosz writes, "Creatures use tools, ornaments, and appliances to augment their bodily capacities. Are their bodies lacking something, which they need to replace with artificial or substitute organs? Or conversely, should prostheses be understood, in terms of aesthetic reorganization and proliferation, as the consequence of an inventiveness that functions beyond and perhaps in defiance of pragmatic need?" Elaine Scarry argues that every artifact recreates and extends the body. Chairs supplement the skeleton, tools append the hands, clothing augments the skin. In Scarry's thinking, "furniture and houses are neither more nor less interior to the human body than the food it absorbs, nor are they fundamentally different from such sophisticated prosthetics as artificial lungs, eyes and kidneys. The consumption of manufactured things turns the body inside out, opening it up *to* and *as* the culture of objects." Mark

Wigley, a professor of architecture, continues this line of thinking about how architecture supplements our natural capabilities, and argues that "a blurring of identity is produced by all prostheses." Some of this work relies on Freud's earlier characterization of man's relation to objects as one of extension.

Medical Imaging

Medical imaging is the visualization of the interior of a body. It is the technique and process which seeks to reveal internal structures for clinical diagnosis, treatment and disease monitoring. There are many types of medical imaging, the main types of imaging used in modern medicine are radiography, magnetic resonance imaging (MRI), nuclear medicine imaging(such as PET and SPECT), and ultrasound.

Commonly used Medical Imaging Methods

Radiography

Radiography uses electromagnetic radiation in X-ray range (ionizing radiation) to take images of the internal parts of the body by sending X-raybeams through the body. The X-rays are absorbed by the material they pass through in differing amounts depending on the density and composition of the material.

Computed Tomography

Computed Tomography (CT) is an imaging technique that combines a series of X-ray images taken from different angles to create cross-sectional internal images, resulting in more detailed images compared to regular X-rays.

Magnetic Resonance Imaging

Magnetic Resonance Imaging (MRI) involves radio waves and magnetic fields to look at the internal structures of the body. The MRI scanner uses powerful magnets to polarize and excite hydrogen nuclei of water molecules, hydrocarbons and other molecules containing hydrogen in human tissue, producing a detectable signal resulting in images of the body.

Nuclear Medicine Scan

Nuclear Medicine Scan (such as PET and SPECT) involves in the use of radioactive tracers, which are radioactive materials that are injected or swallowed to travel through the circulatory or digestive system. The principle behind the use of radioactive tracers is that an atom in a chemical compound is replaced by another atom, of the same chemical element. The substituting atom, however, is a radioactive isotope. This process is often called radioactive labeling. The radiation produced by the tracer can then be detected by the use of a special camera (e.g. gamma camera) to take pictures of tissues and organs in the body to observe its activity and function.

Ultrasound Imaging

Ultrasound Imaging uses high frequency sound waves which are reflected off body tissue to create images of organs, muscles, joints, and other soft tissues. The light travels through the skin layers which can be viewed by using electronic sensors.

Digital Image

A digital image is a numeric representation of a two-dimensional image. Depending on whether the image resolution is fixed, it may be of vector or raster type. By itself, the term "digital image" usually refers to raster images or bitmapped images. Digital images (raster images or bitmapped images) are made of picture elements called Pixels.

Resolution and Size of the Image

Pixels are organized in an ordered rectangular array. The resolution of an image is determined by the dimensions of this pixel array: The image width is the number of columns, and the image height is the number of rows in the array.

Each pixel contains a brightness value. The range of values(how many brightness levels) for each pixel is called color depth and it determines image quality. Each pixel can contain only basic colours or shades of gray which can be typically sufficiently saved in 8 bits (256 values). However the true colour images need 24 bits or more (over 16 milions of colours). The size of the image (e.g. in MB) is then given by: resolution of the image times bits for the pixel (color depth).

Image Digitization

Digitization is the process used to convert analogue data (such as analogue image) into digital form that is saved in the computer memory, through two steps:

1. Sampling

Sampling means dividing the image in pixels. Sampling gives the resolution of a digital image (e.g. in megapixels Mpx). It is necessary to choose an appropriate resolution to preserve all the information that are wanted to be capture.

2. Quantization

Quantization means assigning a numerical value to every pixel. The value represents color (brightness) of the pixel. E.g. 8-bit quantization offers $2^8 = 256$ numerical values for each pixel.

Image Contrast

Contrast can be defined as the differences in intensities of colors between the pixels in an image. If the differences in intensities are high then that translates to an image having a high contrast, but if the differences in intensities were low then the image would have a low contrast.

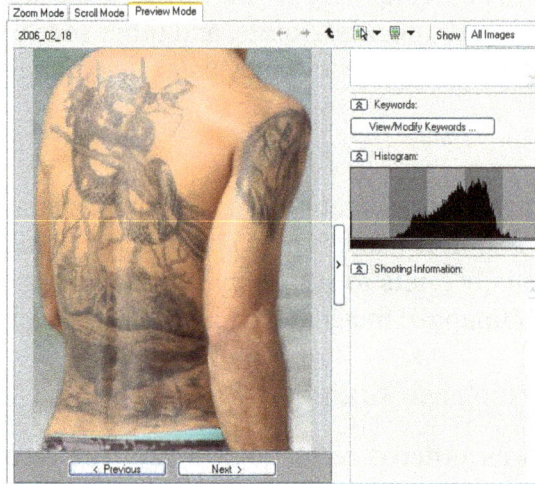

Image Histogram

Image histogram is a graphical representation showing amount of pixels in the image for each brightness value.

Examples of usage of histogram

- Brightness and contrast adjustments
- Equalization of an image
- Thresholding (results in two colours only - black/white)

Image Formats

Some of the more common examples of digital image formats are JPEG, TIFF, GIF and PNG.

Compression

Most of the Digital Image Formats can be divided by their compression method:

- Loseless

No information is lost from the digital image file when a compression algorithm is applied to it. Includes: RAW, TIFF, PNG and BMP. Those image formats store the full

RGB digital image without any loss of information. This comes with the advantage of permitting high quality reproductions but at the price of requiring a lot of memory to save those files.

- Lossy

Results in the loss of some image information to achieve a smaller file size. Includes: JPEG, GIF.

In Pregnancy

Medical imaging may be indicated in pregnancy because of pregnancy complications, intercurrent diseases or routine prenatal care. Magnetic resonance imaging (MRI) without MRI contrast agents as well as obstetric ultrasonography are not associated with any risk for the mother or the fetus, and are the imaging techniques of choice for pregnant women. Projectional radiography, X-ray computed tomography and nuclear medicine imaging result some degree of ionizing radiation exposure, but have with a few exceptions much lower absorbed doses than what are associated with fetal harm. At higher dosages, effects can include miscarriage, birth defects and intellectual disability.

Maximizing Imaging Procedure use

The amount of data obtained in a single MR or CT scan is very extensive. Some of the data that radiologists discard could save patients time and money, while reducing their exposure to radiation and risk of complications from invasive procedures. Another approach for making the procedures more efficient is based on utilizing additional constraints, e.g., in some medical imaging modalities one can improve the efficiency of the data acquisition by taking into account the fact the reconstructed density is positive.

Creation of Three-dimensional Images

Volume rendering techniques have been developed to enable CT, MRI and ultrasound scanning software to produce 3D images for the physician. Traditionally CT and MRI scans produced 2D static output on film. To produce 3D images, many scans are made, then combined by computers to produce a 3D model, which can then be manipulated by the physician. 3D ultrasounds are produced using a somewhat similar technique. In diagnosing disease of the viscera of the abdomen, ultrasound is particularly sensitive on imaging of biliary tract, urinary tract and female reproductive organs (ovary, fallopian tubes). As for example, diagnosis of gallstone by dilatation of common bile duct and stone in the common bile duct. With the ability to visualize important structures in great detail, 3D visualization methods are a valuable resource for the diagnosis and surgical treatment of much pathology. It was a key resource for the famous, but ultimately unsuccessful attempt by Singaporean surgeons to separate Iranian twins Ladan and Laleh Bijani in 2003. The 3D equipment was used previously for similar operations with great success.

Other proposed or developed techniques include:

- Diffuse optical tomography

- Elastography

- Electrical impedance tomography

- Optoacoustic imaging

- Ophthalmology

  - A-scan

  - B-scan

  - Corneal topography

  - Optical coherence tomography

  - Scanning laser ophthalmoscopy

Some of these techniques are still at a research stage and not yet used in clinical routines.

Non-diagnostic Imaging

Neuroimaging has also been used in experimental circumstances to allow people (especially disabled persons) to control outside devices, acting as a brain computer interface.

Many medical imaging software applications (3DSlicer, ImageJ, MIPAV, ImageVis3D, etc.) are used for non-diagnostic imaging, specifically because they don't have an FDA approval and not allowed to use in clinical research for patient diagnosis. Note that many clinical research studies are not designed for patient diagnosis anyway.

Archiving and Recording

Used primarily in ultrasound imaging, capturing the image produced by a medical imaging device is required for archiving and telemedicine applications. In most scenarios, a frame grabber is used in order to capture the video signal from the medical device and relay it to a computer for further processing and operations.

DICOM

The Digital Imaging and Communication in Medicine (DICOM) Standard is used globally to store, exchange, and transmit medical images. The DICOM Standard incorporates protocols for imaging techniques such as radiography, computed tomography (CT), magnetic resonance imaging (MRI), ultrasonography, and radiation therapy. DICOM includes standards for image exchange (e.g., via portable media such as DVDs), image compression, 3-D visualization, image presentation, and results reporting.

Compression of Medical Images

Medical imaging techniques produce very large amounts of data, especially from CT, MRI and PET modalities. As a result, storage and communications of electronic image data are prohibitive without the use of compression. JPEG 2000 is the state-of-the-art image compression DICOM standard for storage and transmission of medical images. The cost and feasibility of accessing large image data sets over low or various bandwidths are further addressed by use of another DICOM standard, called JPIP, to enable efficient streaming of the JPEG 2000 compressed image data.

Medical Imaging in the Cloud

There has been growing trend to migrate from PACS to a Cloud Based RIS. A recent article by Applied Radiology said, "As the digital-imaging realm is embraced across the healthcare enterprise, the swift transition from terabytes to petabytes of data has put radiology on the brink of information overload. Cloud computing offers the imaging department of the future the tools to manage data much more intelligently."

Use in Pharmaceutical Clinical Trials

Medical imaging has become a major tool in clinical trials since it enables rapid diagnosis with visualization and quantitative assessment.

A typical clinical trial goes through multiple phases and can take up to eight years. Clinical endpoints or outcomes are used to determine whether the therapy is safe and effective. Once a patient reaches the endpoint, he or she is generally excluded from further experimental interaction. Trials that rely solely on clinical endpoints are very costly as they have long durations and tend to need large numbers of patients.

In contrast to clinical endpoints, surrogate endpoints have been shown to cut down the time required to confirm whether a drug has clinical benefits. Imaging biomarkers (a characteristic that is objectively measured by an imaging technique, which is used as an indicator of pharmacological response to a therapy) and surrogate endpoints have shown to facilitate the use of small group sizes, obtaining quick results with good statistical power.

Imaging is able to reveal subtle change that is indicative of the progression of therapy that may be missed out by more subjective, traditional approaches. Statistical bias is reduced as the findings are evaluated without any direct patient contact.

Imaging techniques such as positron emission tomography (PET) and magnetic resonance imaging (MRI) are routinely used in oncology and neuroscience areas,. For example, measurement of tumour shrinkage is a commonly used surrogate endpoint in solid tumour response evaluation. This allows for faster and more objective assessment of the effects of anticancer drugs. In Alzheimer's disease, MRI scans of the entire brain can accurately assess the rate of hippocampal atrophy , while PET scans can measure the brain's metabolic activity by measuring regional glucose metabolism, and beta-amyloid plaques using tracers such as Pittsburgh compound B (PiB). Historically less use has been made of quantitative medical imaging in other areas of drug development although interest is growing.

An imaging-based trial will usually be made up of three components:

1. A realistic imaging protocol. The protocol is an outline that standardizes (as far as practically possible) the way in which the images are acquired using the various modalities. It covers the specifics in which images are to be stored, processed and evaluated.

2. An imaging center that is responsible for collecting the images, perform quality control and provide tools for data storage, distribution and analysis. It is important for images acquired at different time points are displayed in a standardized format to maintain the reliability of the evaluation. Certain specialized imaging contract research organizations provide end to end medical imaging services, from protocol design and site management through to data quality assurance and image analysis.

3. Clinical sites that recruit patients to generate the images to send back to the imaging center.

Shielding

Lead is the main material used for radiographic shielding against scattered X-rays.

In magnetic resonance imaging, there is MRI RF shielding as well as magnetic shielding to prevent external disturbance of image quality.

Algebraic Reconstruction Technique

In Computed Tomography (CT), three dimensional reconstruction techniques from projection have been used for many years in radiology. The two dimensional Fourier transform is the most commonly used algorithm in radiology. In this technique a large number of projections at uniformly distributed angles around the subject are required for reconstruction of the image. The Algebraic Reconstruction Technique uses three or more projections to reconstruct the 2-dimensional beam density distribution.

The ART algorithms have a simple intuitive basis. Each projected density is thrown back across the reconstruction space in which the densities are iteratively modified to bring each reconstructed projection into agreement with the measured projection. Assuming that the pattern being reconstructed is enclosed in a square space of n x n array of small pixels ρ_j $\left(j = 1,...,n^2 \right)$ is grayness or density number, which is uniform within the pixel but different from other pixels. A "ray" is a region of the square space which lies between two parallel lines. The weighted ray sum is the total grayness of the reconstruction figure within the ray. The projection at a given angle is then the sum of non-overlapping, equally wide rays covering the figure. The ART algorithm consists of altering the grayness of each pixel intersected by the ray in such a way as to make the ray sum agree with the corresponding element of the measured projection. Assume **P** is a matrix of m xn^2 and the m component column vector R. Let $p_{i,j}$ denote the (i,j)th element of P, and R_i denote the ith ray of the reconstructed projection vector $_2$R. For $1 \leq i \leq m$ N_i is number of pixels under projection ray R$_i$, defined as $N_i = \sum_{j=1}^{n^2} p_{i,j}^2$. ART is an iterative method. The density number ρ_j^q denotes the value of ρ_j after q iterations. After q iterations the intensity of the ith reconstructed projection ray is

$$R_i^q = \sum_{j=1}^{n^2} p_{i,j}\, p_j^q\,,$$

And the density in each pixel is

$$\rho_j^{\sim q+1} = \rho_j^q + p_{i,j}\frac{R_i - R_i^q}{N_i}, \text{ with starting value } \rho_j^{\sim 0} = 0$$

Where R_i is the measured projection ray and

$$i = \begin{cases} m, \text{ if } (q+1) \text{ is divisible} \\ \text{the remainder of dividing } (q+1) \text{ by m, otherwis} \end{cases}$$

and,

$$\rho_j^q = \begin{cases} 0, & \text{if } \rho^{\sim q} \leq 0 \\ \rho_j^{\sim q}, & \text{if } 0 \leq p_j^{\sim q} \leq 1 \\ 1, & \text{if } \rho_j^{\sim q} \geq 1 \end{cases}$$

This algorithm is known as fully constrained ART.

It is necessary to determine when an iterative algorithm has converged to a solution which is optimal according to some criterion. Various criteria for convergence have been devised. The discrepancy between the measured and calculated projection elements is

$$D^q \equiv \left\{ \frac{1}{m} \sum_{i=1}^{m} \frac{(R_i - R_i^q)^2}{N_i} \right\}^{\frac{1}{2}},$$

And the nonuniformity or variance of constructed figure is

$$V^q \equiv \sum_j \left(\rho_j^q - \overline{\rho}\right)^2,$$

And the entropy constructed figure

$$E^q \equiv \frac{-1}{2\log n} \sum_j \left(\frac{\rho_j^q}{\overline{\rho}}\right) \log \left(\frac{\rho_j^q}{\overline{\rho}}\right).$$

D^q tends to zero, V^q to a minimum and S^q to a maximum with increasing q. For a known test pattern $\left(\rho_{i,j}^t\right)$, the Euclidean Distance is define as

$$S^q \equiv \sqrt{\frac{1}{n^2} \sum_j \left(\rho_j^q - \rho_j^t\right)^2}.$$

Dual-energy X-ray Absorptiometry

Dual-energy x-ray absorptiometry (DEXA) is the technique of choice in the assessment of bone mineral density (BMD), the average concentration of mineral in a defined section of bone. DEXA is a quick method that is accurate (exact measurement of BMD), precise (reproducible), and flexible (different regions can be scanned) and is performed with a low radiation dose. Although other factors, such as trabecular bone structure, are important, central BMD measurements are helpful in the diagnosis of osteoporosis for estimating the risk of nontraumatic fracture and in choosing and monitoring treatments. Understanding every step of the procedure is important for maximizing the usefulness of the imaging evaluation to patients and referring clinicians.

A DEXA scanner consists of a low-dose x-ray tube with two energies for separating mineral and soft-tissue components and a high-resolution multidetector array. The devices have one of two different systems: a fan-beam device that emits alternating high (140 kVp) and low (70–100 kVp) x-rays and sweeps across a scan area or a constant x-ray beam with a rare-earth filter and energy-specific absorption, which separates photons of higher (70 keV) and lower (40 keV) energy.

Image Acquisition

Areas Scanned

In adult patients, central DEXA measurements of the lumbar spine and proximal femur are recommended. Two regions should be measured so that if one is unavailable, the forearm can be imaged. For children (younger than 20 years) only the lumbar spine is studied because variability in femoral maturation results in lack of reproducibility in the hip region, so the reference database is available only for the spine.

Lumbar spine—Posteroanterior images of the lumbar spine include vertebral bodies L1–L4.

Proximal femur—either hip may be used for DEXA of the proximal femur. The lowest-level data on the femoral neck and total hip are used for diagnosis. Total hip is the most reproducible measurement of the hip.

Forearm—the forearm is used in three conditions when the hip and spine cannot be measured or the data interpreted, in examinations of patients with hyperparathyroidism and those whose weight exceeds the limit for the table. Primary hyperparathyroidism decreases BMD, which is greater in structures with predominantly cortical bone as opposed to trabecular bone. Recommendations include measurement at the three sites (hip, spine, and radius) for diagnosis and for follow-up after surgical and medical treatment. The areas imaged are total bone, one third of the radius, the ultradistal radius, and the ulna. The most useful measurements are the ultradistal portion of the radius as an indicator of trabecular bone loss and the distal one third of the radius (distal radial diaphysis, excluding the ultradistal portion) as an indicator of cortical bone mineral loss.

Appropriate Patient Positioning

Appropriate patient positioning is essential for optimizing BMD measurement. The patients are placed in the supine position for posteroanterior imaging of the lumbar spine and femoral neck and sitting next to the table for imaging of the forearm.

Image Assessment

Images are assessed for patient movement. The area of interest exceeding 1–2 cm and superior and inferior limits should be included to verify that the complete anatomic region is scanned. The bone axis should be straight and centered, and the lesser trochanter should not be seen on images of the proximal femur.

Analysis

Placement of Region of Interest

Equipment from various manufacturers generates automatic ROIs, which should be reviewed. Correct numbering of vertebral bodies is the main goal in DEXA of the lumbar spine. The indicators of correct positioning are as follows: the ribs appear at T12, the largest transverse processes are L3, the vertebral area values increase from L1 to L4, BMD increases from L1 to L3, and the BMD of L4 is similar to or slightly less than that of L3. Sometimes radiographs are necessary for correlation. Altered vertebrae (deformed or with lesions or artifacts in them) should be excluded from the analysis. If only one vertebral body is left, the region is not useful for diagnosis. In hip scanning, it is important to avoid undesired bone. The anatomic landmark selected for femoral neck ROI placement is the greater trochanteric notch.

Pitfalls

Inappropriate patient positioning—The most important source of false BMD measurements is inappropriate patient positioning. Longitudinal in vivo precision reflects variability due to positioning: spine, 1.1%; femoral neck, 1.2%; trochanter 1.3%.

Artifacts—Images should be assessed for artifacts, which should be excluded from the ROI. Artifacts include dense objects such as piercings, catheters, and surgical material; retained contrast medium, such as barium and myelographic agents; and vertebroplasty cement. Calcifications that do not affect the analysis, such as calcified kidneys, hydatid cysts, myomas, and lithiasis, should be noted in the report as incidental findings. Calcifications superimposed on the ROI, such as dermatomyositis and bone grafts, should be noted as causes of increased BMD.

Disorders—Many diseases spuriously alter BMD measurement. In analysis of the lumbar spine, a greater than 1 point difference in T-score between two adjacent vertebrae indicates a vertebra is abnormal, and radiography is mandatory for diagnosis. Degeneration due to osteoarthrosis artifactually increases spinal BMD in elderly patients and causes several morphologic changes, such as osteophytes (bone growths) and vertebral endplate reactions to degenerative disks. In the presence of fractures, BMD is altered owing to higher bone density with a smaller surface. Lytic and sclerotic bone lesions, such as metastatic lesions, lymphoma, bone islands, lesions due to Paget disease, hemangiomas, and dense pedicles, also are impediments to BMD measurement. Diffuse diseases, such as ankylosing spondylitis and osteopetrosis, alter osseous structure and bone density.

Interpretation

The scanner calculates BMD in grams per square centimeter. A reference database is consulted, and values and curves are obtained. The main parameters are T-score, which represents the SD by which the BMD differs from the mean BMD of a young adult reference population of the same ethnicity and sex, and Z-score, which is the SD by which the BMD differs from the mean BMD of a healthy population of the same ethnicity, sex, and age as the person undergoing DEXA.

Tomography

Tomography is a radiologic technique for obtaining clear X-ray images of deep internal structures by focusing on a specific plane within the body. Structures that are obscured by overlying organs and soft tissues that are insufficiently delineated on conventional X rays can thus be adequately visualized.

The simplest method is linear tomography, in which the X-ray tube is moved in a straight line in one direction while the film moves in the opposite direction. As these shifts occur, the X-ray tube continues to emit radiation so that most structures in the part of the body under examination are blurred by motion. Only those objects lying in a plane coinciding with the pivot point of a line between the tube and the film are in focus. A somewhat more complicated technique known as multidirectional tomography produces an even sharper image by moving the film and X-ray tube in a circular or elliptical pattern. As long as both tube and film move in synchrony, a clear image of objects in the focal plane can be produced. These tomographic approaches have been used to study the kidneys and other abdominal structures that are surrounded by tissues of nearly the same density and so cannot be differentiated by conventional X-ray techniques. They have also been employed to examine the small bones and other structures of the ear, which are surrounded by relatively dense temporal bone.

A still more complex technique, variously called computerized tomography (CT), or computerized axial tomography (CAT), was developed by Godfrey Hounsfield of Great Britain and Allen Cormack of the United States during the early 1970s. Since then it has become a widely used diagnostic approach. In this procedure a narrow beam of X rays sweeps across an area of the body and is recorded not on film but by a radiation detector as a pattern of electrical impulses. Data from many such sweeps are integrated by a computer, which uses the radiation absorption figures to assess the density of tissues at thousands of points. The density values appear on a television-like screen as points of varying brightness to produce a detailed cross-sectional image of the internal structure under scrutiny.

Synchrotron X-ray Tomographic Microscopy

A new technique called synchrotron X-ray tomographic microscopy (SRXTM) allows for detailed three-dimensional scanning of fossils.

The construction of third-generation synchrotron sources combined with the tremendous improvement of detector technology, data storage and processing capabilities since the 1990s has led to a boost of high-end synchrotron tomography in materials research with a wide range of different applications, e.g. the visualization and quantitative analysis of differently absorbing phases, microporosities, cracks, precipitates or grains in a specimen. Synchrotron radiation is created by accelerating free particles in high vacuum. By the laws of electrodynamics this acceleration leads to the emission of electromagnetic radiation (Jackson, 1975). Linear particle acceleration is one possibility, but apart from the very high electric fields one would need it is more practical to hold the charged particles on a closed trajectory in order to obtain a source of continuous radiation. Magnetic fields are used to force the particles onto the desired orbit and prevent them from flying in a straight line. The radial acceleration associated with the change of direction then generates radiation.

Volume Rendering

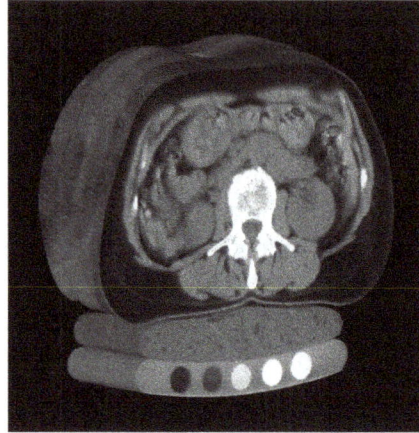

Figure: Multiple X-ray computed tomographs (with quantitative mineral density calibration) stacked to form a 3D model.

Volume rendering is a set of techniques used to display a 2D projection of a 3D discretely sampled data set, typically a 3D scalar field. A typical 3D data set is a group of 2D slice images acquired, for example, by a CT, MRI, or MicroCT scanner. These are usually acquired in a regular pattern (e.g., one slice every millimeter) and usually have a regular number of image pixels in a regular pattern. This is an example of a regular volumetric grid, with each volume element, or voxel represented by a single value that is obtained by sampling the immediate area surrounding the voxel.

To render a 2D projection of the 3D data set, one first needs to define a camera in space relative to the volume. Also, one needs to define the opacity and color of every voxel. This is usually defined using an RGBA (for red, green, blue, alpha) transfer function that defines the RGBA value for every possible voxel value.

For example, a volume may be viewed by extracting isosurfaces (surfaces of equal values) from the volume and rendering them as polygonal meshes or by rendering the volume directly as a block of data. The marching cubes algorithm is a common technique for extracting an isosurface from volume data. Direct volume rendering is a computationally intensive task that may be performed in several ways.

Functional Imaging

Functional imaging is a techniques to study of human brain function based on analysis of data acquired using brain imaging modalities such as Electroencephalography

(EEG), Magnetoencephalography (MEG), functional Magnetic Resonance Imaging (fMRI), Positron Emission Tomography (PET) or Optical Imaging.

Modern functional imaging has two main advantages over the multi/single-unit recordings used to study the electrophysiology of neurons. The first is that it is generally non-invasive, and is therefore applicable routinely in humans. This allows for the study of unique human attributes such as language. The second is that it can provide a wide field of view. Rather than recording information about a single or small number of neuronal cells, an image may be gathered summarizing simultaneous activity across the whole brain. This provides a different yet complementary perspective on neural coding. A disadvantage, however, is that functional imaging provides only an indirect measure of the quantities of primary interest to neuroscientists e.g., firing rates and membrane potentials. Current research is aimed at bridging this gap using a combination of experimental and mathematical modelling approaches.

Modalities

Current imaging modalities include the Electroencephalogram (EEG) which records electrical voltages from electrodes placed on the scalp and the Magnetoencephalogram (MEG) which records the magnetic field from SQUID sensors placed above the head. Both MEG and EEG have a high temporal resolution (milliseconds), capable of detecting e.g., the 40Hz Gamma response implicated in object representation. Their spatial resolution is, however, usually of the order of centimeters rather than millimeters. This varies a great deal, depending on the nature of the neuronal activity one is trying to localize. It depends in particular on the number of sources that is activated at the time data is recorded. In practice this implies that e.g. for isolating subtle cognitive components, a lower resolution is to be expected, whilst the stronger early components of an auditory response can be localized to within millimeters in the brainstem.

In contrast, functional Magnetic Resonance Imaging (fMRI) has low temporal (hundreds of milliseconds or seconds) but relatively high spatial (millimeters) resolution. Increases in neural activity cause variations in blood oxygenation, which in turn cause magnetization changes that can be detected in an MRI scanner. This Blood Oxygenation Level Dependent (BOLD) signal peaks up to 6s after neuronal activity. Moreover, the hemodynamics act like a low pass filter , smearing out changes in local electrical activity.

Simultaneous recordings of EEG and fMRI (Ritter and Villringer, 2006) have the potential to localize neuronal activity with both high temporal and spatial resolution. Other important imaging modalities are PET and Optical Imaging. PET's spatial resolution typically falls somewhere between that of fMRI and MEG/EEG. In addition, PET has very low temporal resolution (tens of seconds to minutes) and requires injection of a trace amount of radioactivity. This limits the number of measurements that can be made on any one individual. But a great advantage of PET is that it is particularly useful in the study of brain neurophysiology and neurochemistry e.g., one can image glucose uptake and the activity at serotonin and dopamine receptors, in systems of importance to those studying anxiety, depression and addiction. Optical Imaging or Near Infrared Spectroscopy (NIRs) can also detect BOLD signals from changes in the amount of reflected light. This is an economical alternative to fMRI but is limited to imaging the cortex.

Functional imaging is also closely related to structural imaging, in which MRI is used to provide high resolution images with high contrast between *e.g.,* white matter and gray matter. (DTI) which can show the direction of white matter fibres.

Functional Specialization

There are two key themes in the analysis of functional imaging data. They reflect the long-standing debate in neuroscience about functional specialization versus functional integration in the brain (Cohen and Tong, 2001). The first is brain `mapping' where three-dimensional images of neuronal activation are produced showing which parts of the brain respond to a given cognitive or sensory challenge. This is also known as the study of functional specialization and generally proceeds using some form of Statistical Parametric Mapping (SPM). A classic example here is the identification of human V4 and V5, the areas specialized for the processing of color and motion.

SPM is a voxel-based approach, employing classical statistics and topological inference, to make comments about regionally specific responses to experimental factors. PET or fMRI data are first spatially processed so that they conform to a known anatomical space, in which responses are, characterized statistically typically using the General Linear Model (GLM). For fMRI data the GLM embodies a convolution model of the hemodynamic response. This accounts for the fact that BOLD signals are a delayed and dispersed version of the neuronal response. GLMs are fitted at each voxel and inferences are made about which parts of the brain are active, in a statistical sense. To accommodate the spatial nature of the imaging data (and account for the multiple statistical comparisons made) SPM techniques make use of Random Field Theory (RFT) and/or other statistical procedures, e.g., False Discovery Rate.

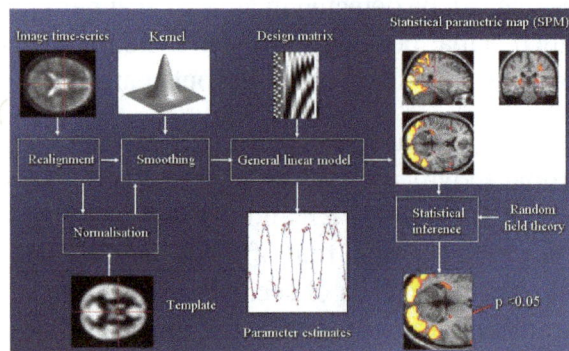

Figure: Processing stream for brain mapping using PET or fMRI data

The SPM approach can also be used with structural data to find brain regions containing a higher gray matter density. This is known as Voxel-Based Morphometry (VBM) and has been used, for example, to show that the posterior hippocampus, useful for spatial navigation, is enlarged in taxi drivers.

For MEG or EEG, data can be analyzed in sensor space, furnishing a crude spatial mapping of brain function. Functions can, however, be more accurately localized using source reconstruction methods. These work by specifying a forward model describing how a current source in the brain propagates to become an MEG or EEG measurement, using Maxwell's equations. These models are then inverted using statistical inference. Data from sensory systems is often analyzed using an averaging procedure. The data immediately following a sensory event, *e.g.*, hearing an auditory tone, is averaged over multiple events to produce an Event Related Potential (ERP). Components of the ERP can then be localized to different parts of the brain. Other cognitive components, however, are not easily isolated using this ERP approach. For these, a time-frequency characterization may be more appropriate.

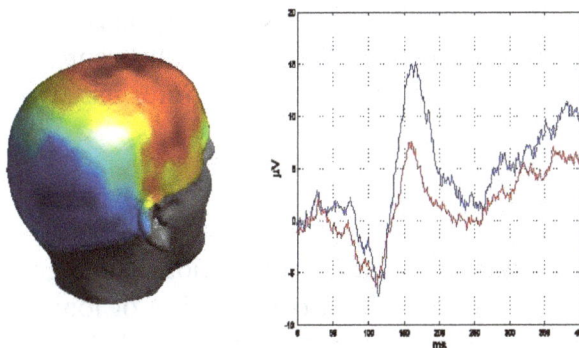

Figure: Sensor distribution of EEG at a single time point and ERPs for two different experimental conditions

Functional Integration

The second theme is 'functional integration', where models are used to describe how different brain areas interact. A classic example is the use of models to find increased connectivity between dorsal and ventral visual streams after subjects learn object-place associations. A wide range of statistical techniques are being used to measure inter-regional connectivity. Both unsupervised (e.g., Independent Component Analysis, ICA) and supervised techniques (e.g., support vector machine, SVM) are used. Other models seek to directly measure "causal" connectivity based on static, statistical constraints (e.g., Structural Equation Modelling, SEM) or dynamic, more bio-physically motivated assumptions (e.g., Dynamic Causal Modelling, DCM). A challenge for functional integration models is to bridge the gap between the large-scale, statistical models of the whole brain, and the small number of highly constrained spatial regions needed to be able to apply SEM and/or DCM.

DCM for fMRI uses a forward model in which neural activity generates BOLD signal changes via a `Balloon' model of vascular dynamics. The model is then inverted to provide estimates of changes in connectivity between brain regions. In DCM for ERPs, neural activity is described using neural-mass models, which then give rise to observed EEG or MEG data using Maxwell's equations. Inversion of the model then allows one to make inferences about changes in long-range excitatory connections among different brain areas.

Radiology

Radiology represents a branch of medicine that deals with radiant energy in the diagnosis and treatment of diseases. This field can be divided into two broad areas – diagnostic radiology and interventional radiology. A physician who specializes in radiology is called radiologist.

The outcome of an imaging study does not rely merely on the indication or the quality of its technical execution. Diagnostic radiology specialist represents the last link in the diagnostic chain, as they search for relevant image information to evaluate and finally support a sound diagnosis.

Radiology Techniques

Similar to the images produced in 1895, conventional radiographic images (usually shortened to X-rays) are produced by a combination of ionizing radiation (without added contrast materials such as barium or iodine) and light striking a photosensitive surface, which in turn produces a latent image that is subsequently processed.

The major advantages of conventional radiography are relative inexpensiveness of the images and the possibility to obtain them virtually anywhere by using mobile or portable machines (for example, mammography). Disadvantages are the limited range of densities it can demonstrate and the use of ionizing radiation.

Computed tomography (CT) currently represents the workhorse of radiology. Recent developments permit extremely fast volume scans that can generate two-dimensional slices in all possible orientations, as well as sophisticated three-dimensional reconstructions. Nevertheless, the radiation dose remains high, thus a very strict indication for every intended CT is needed.

Ultrasonography is still the cheapest and most harmless technology in radiology, which is the reason why many physicians outside radiology use this technique. Ultrasound probes utilize acoustic energy above the audible frequency of humans in order to produce images. As there is no ionizing radiation with this modality, it is particularly useful in imaging of children and pregnant women.

Magnetic resonance imaging (MRI) makes use of the potential energy stored in the body's hydrogen atoms. Those atoms are manipulated by very strong magnetic fields and radiofrequency pulses to produce adequate amount of localizing and tissue-specific energy that will be used by highly sophisticated computer programs in order to generate two-dimensional and three-dimensional images. The major advantage is that no ionizing radiation is used.

Fluoroscopy represents a modality where X-rays are used in performing real-time visualization of the body, allowing for evaluation of body parts, administered contrast flow and positioning changes of bones and joints. Radiation doses in fluoroscopy are substantially higher when compared to conventional radiography, as many images are acquired for every minute of the procedure.

Nuclear medicine images are made by giving the patient a short-lived radioactive material, and then using gamma camera or positron emission scanner that records radiation emanating from the patient. Most common nuclear medicine modalities used in clinical practice are single-photon emission computed tomography (SPECT) and positron emission tomography (PET).

Finally, advances in equipment and increases in computer power have allowed combining data imaging sets from various modalities in radiology; the most popular use of this has been integration of PET functional nuclear medicine data with CT anatomic data (PET/CT), which currently has widespread use in the imaging of cancer.

Interventional Radiology

Interventional radiology (IR or sometimes VIR for vascular and interventional radiology) is a subspecialty of radiology in which minimally invasive procedures are performed using image guidance. Some of these procedures are done for purely diagnostic purposes (e.g., angiogram), while others are done for treatment purposes (e.g., angioplasty).

The basic concept behind interventional radiology is to diagnose or treat pathologies, with the most minimally invasive technique possible. Minimally invasive procedures are currently performed more than ever before. These procedures are often performed with the patient fully awake, with little or no sedation required. Interventional Radiologists and Interventional Radiographers diagnose and treat several disorders, including peripheral vascular disease, renal artery stenosis, inferior vena cava filter placement, gastrostomy tube placements, biliary stents and hepatic interventions. Images are used for guidance, and the primary instruments used during the procedure are needles and catheters. The images provide maps that allow the Clinician to guide these instruments through the body to the areas containing disease. By minimizing the physical trauma to the patient, peripheral interventions can reduce infection rates and recovery times, as well as hospital stays. To be a trained interventionalist in the United States, an individual completes a five-year residency in radiology and a one- or two-year fellowship in IR.

Analysis of Images

Teleradiology

Teleradiology is the transmission of radiographic images from one location to another for interpretation by an appropriately trained professional, usually a Radiologist or Reporting Radiographer. It is most often used to allow rapid interpretation of emergency room, ICU and other emergent examinations after hours of usual operation, at night and on weekends. In these cases, the images can be sent across time zones (e.g. to Spain, Australia, India) with the receiving Clinician working his normal daylight hours. However at present, large private teleradiology companies in the U.S. currently provide most after-hours coverage employing night working Radiologists in the U.S. Teleradiology can also be used to obtain consultation with an expert or subspecialist about a complicated or puzzling case.

Teleradiology requires a sending station, a high-speed internet connection, and a high-quality receiving station. At the transmission station, plain radiographs are passed through a digitizing machine before transmission, while CT, MRI, ultrasound and nuclear medicine scans can be sent directly, as they are already digital data. The computer at the receiving end will need to have a high-quality display screen that has been tested and cleared for clinical purposes. Reports are then transmitted to the requesting clinician.

The major advantage of teleradiology is the ability to use different time zones to provide real-time emergency radiology services around-the-clock. The disadvantages include higher costs, limited contact between the referrer and the reporting Clinician, and the inability to cover for procedures requiring an onsite reporting Clinician. Laws and regulations concerning the use of teleradiology vary among the states, with some requiring a license to practice medicine in the state sending the radiologic exam. In the U.S., some states require the teleradiology report to be preliminary with the official report issued by a hospital staff Radiologist.

Artificial Intelligence

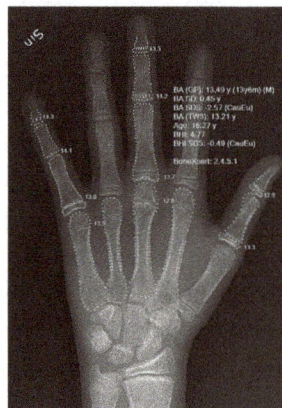

Figure: X-ray of a hand, with automatic calculation of bone age by computer software.

Existing AI systems can outperform radiologists on many diagnostic tasks, and as of 2017, AI systems are continuing to rapidly advance. Many economists and AI researchers believe that most tasks that consist of visually interpreting medical images are likely to be automated in the near future.

Photoacoustic Imaging

Photoacoustic imaging is based on the photoacoustic effect, is a noninvasive imaging modality Optical and rf waves, instead of electromagnetic waves at other wavelengths, are used in photoacoustic imaging because of their desirable physical properties such as deeper tissue penetration and better absorption by contrast agents. The combination of high ultrasonic resolution with good image contrast due to optical/rf absorption is quite advantageous for imaging purposes. When compared with optical imaging, in which the scattering in tissues limits the spatial resolution with increasing depth, photoacoustic imaging has higher spatial resolution and deeper imaging depth since scattering of the ultrasonic signal in tissue is much weaker. When compared with ultrasound imaging, in which the contrast is limited due to the mechanical properties of biological tissues, photoacoustic imaging has better tissue contrast which is related to the optical properties of different tissues. In addition, the absence of ionizing radiation also makes photoacoustic imaging safer than other imaging techniques such as computed tomography and radionuclide-based imaging techniques.

Photoacoustic imaging systems can be briefly categorized into two types: photoacoustic tomography (PAT, also referred to as optoacoustic tomography or thermoacoustic tomography) and photoacoustic microscopy (PAM). Although PAM has gained significant attention over the last several years , we will primarily focus on PAT in this chapter due to spatial limitation. Both non-targeted and molecularly-targeted photoacoustic imaging will be discussed in the following text.

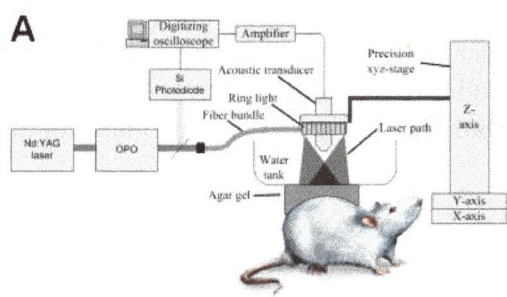

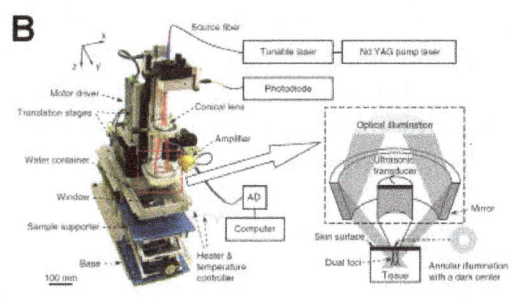

Photoacoustic tomography   **Photoacoustic microscopy**

Figure: Typical setups for photoacoustic tomography (**A**) and photoacoustic microscopy (**B**). Reprinted with permission from .

Contrast Agents For Photoacoustic Imaging

An ideal scenario for photoacoustic imaging would be that light absorption of normal tissue should be low for deeper signal penetration, while the absorption for the object of interest should be high for optimal image contrast . The contrast agents used for photoacoustic imaging can be categorized into two types: endogenous and exogenous contrast agents. Certain endogenous molecules, such as hemoglobin and melanin, have much stronger light absorption than the normal tissue in both the visible and near-infrared (700–900 nm) region. Two of the biggest advantages of using endogenous contrast agents for imaging applications are safety and the possibility to reveal the true "physiological" condition, since the physiological parameters do not change during image acquisition if a relatively slow biological process is imaged.

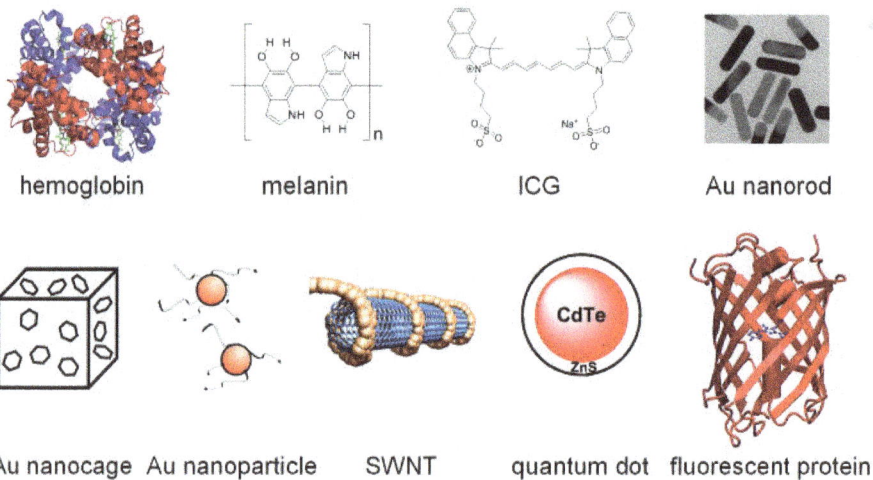

Figure : A wide variety of contrast agents can be used for photoacoustic imaging applications.

In many scenarios such as the detection of early stage tumors, endogenous contrast agent alone is not sufficient to provide useful information. Since the intensity of photoacoustic signal in biological tissue is proportional to optical energy absorption, which is proportional to the amount of the contrast agent , exogenous contrast agents are frequently needed to provide better signal/contrast for photoacoustic imaging. Commonly used contrast agents for photoacoustic imaging include: indocyanine green (ICG), various gold nanoparticles , single-walled carbon nanotubes (SWNTs) , quantum dots (QDs) and fluorescent proteins.

Non-Targeted Photoacoustic Imaging

To date, photoacoustic imaging has generally been used in preclinical research and animal studies. Although none of these studies uses any targeting moiety, with the assistance of proper contrast agents, photoacoustic imaging could be used in many aspects of biomedical research.

Photoacoustic Imaging with Hemoglobin and/or Melanin

Hemoglobin and melanin are the two most important naturally-occurring contrast agents for enhanced photoacoustic imaging. As an endogenous contrast agent, hemoglobin has been explored for photoacoustic imaging in a number of experimental scenarios such as visualizing the brain structure/lesions , imaging small animals , as well as measuring microvascular blood flow.

References

- Wong, J.Y.; Bronzino, J.D.; Peterson, D.R., eds. (2012). Biomaterials: Principles and Practices. Boca Raton, Florida: CRC Press. p. 281. ISBN 9781439872512. Retrieved 12 March 2016

- Ibrahim, H.; Esfahani, S. N.; Poorganji, B.; Dean, D.; Elahinia, M. (January 2017). "Resorbable bone fixation alloys, forming, and post-fabrication treatments". Materials Science and Engineering: C. 70 (1): 870–888. doi:10.1016/j.msec.2016.09.069

- Prosthesis, science: britannica.com, Retrieved 30 June 2018

- "Chapter 1, Part 2, Section 160.19: Phrenic Nerve Stimulator". Medicare National Coverage Determinations Manual (PDF). Centers for Medicare and Medicaid Services. 27 March 2015. Retrieved 19 February 2016

- Wagenberg, B.; Froum, S.J. (2006). "A retrospective study of 1925 consecutively placed immediate implants from 1988 to 2004". The International Journal of Oral & Maxillofacial Implants. 21 (1): 71–80. PMID 16519184

- Tomography, science: britannica.com, Retrieved 25 May 2018

- Duke, J.; Barhan, S. (2007). "Chapter 27: Modern Concepts in Intrauterine Devices". In Falcone, T.; Hurd, W. Clinical Reproductive Medicine and Surgery. Elsevier Health Sciences. pp. 405–416. ISBN 9780323076593. Retrieved 12 March 2016

- Simmons M, Montague D (2008). "Penile prosthesis implantation: past, present, and future". International Journal of Impotence Research. 20: 437–444. doi:10.1038/ijir.2008.11

- Functional-imaging: scholarpedia.org, Retrieved 15 March 2018

- Syring, G. (6 May 2003). "Overview: FDA Regulation of Medical Devices". Quality and Regulatory Associates, LLC. Retrieved 12 March 2016

- Polikov, Vadim S.; Patrick A. Tresco & William M. Reichert (2005). "Response of brain tissue to chronically implanted neural electrodes". Journal of Neuroscience Methods. 148(1): 1–18. doi:10.1016/j.jneumeth.2005.08.015

- What-is-Radiology, health: news-medical.net, Retrieved 10 May 2018

Permissions

Index

www.ingramcontent.com/pod-product-compliance
Lightning Source LLC
Chambersburg PA
CBHW080242230326
41458CB00096B/2919